# Lupus- In Spite of the Wolf

### By: Antonia DiBona

*I'd like to thank the community of people who made this piece possible. I'd like to thank Dr. Stefania Gallucci and her lab at Temple University for letting me see a glimpse into their day to day lives. I'd like to thank Dr. Philip Cohen's lab for inviting me to experience their lab as well. I'd like to thank Erin Castaldi for opening my eyes to the reality of living with lupus every day. I'd like to thank my mother for her always being available to listen to the latest drafts and my father for his never failing support. And finally I'd like to thank the readers for supporting a worthwhile cause. A portion of the proceeds of this book will go towards lupus research.*

**LUPUS-IN SPITE OF THE WOLF**

**TABLE OF CONTENTS**

**1. ERIN CASTALDI** 1

**2. THE LAB** 5

**3. THE LITERARY SIDE** 13

**4. WHEN THINGS WENT WRONG** 17

**5. THE GALLUCCI/CARICCHIO FORCE** 22

**6. TIBETAN LION ON FLOWERS** 32

**7. HER ADVENTUROUS SIDE** 36

**8. THE LFA** 40

**9. IT TAKES TWO** 50

**10. ANNETTE AND CHERI – DEDICATED TO THE LFA** 55

**11. FUNDING PROBLEMS** 61

**12. AN UNWELCOME GOODBYE** 66

**13. FEELING THE EFFECTS OF DWINDLING FUNDS** 69

**14. DISCOVERIES** 74

**15. BEATING THE ODDS** 78

**REFLECTION** 85

# 1. Erin Castaldi

Dear Diary, 1-14-06

It has become achingly obvious that this disease of mine will not let go. I need to surrender, somewhat[,] my pride and will to working with the malice, not against it. – Erin Castaldi

\*\*\*

She felt like a speck. An inconsequential speck. What could she offer anyone? She couldn't even offer anything to herself. She was just another sick person, living off of government help because she couldn't afford the medication that only slightly lessened the pain she was in. She felt guilty. Guilty about not being a better wife. Guilty about needing government assistance. Guilty about not being a better citizen and not giving back anything to society. She viewed herself as a taker and she wanted so badly to be a giver.

She had time to dwell on concepts like purpose and what's it all about. She had so much time, that time almost drove her mad. She tried to find hobbies and things to do for a person who was chronically sick. Watching movie after movie borrowed from the local library wasn't cutting it. She had tried a part time job, but it proved too much. So she thought she'd get her yoga instructing certificate, but the disease butchered that process as well and made carnage of her body. To pass the time she joined a pen pal program where she got assigned a pen pal who was in prison. In some small way, she could relate. Her body was like a prison unto itself.

\*\*\*\*

When I first met Erin, she sat in the corner of the coffee shop in the comfy chairs by the window. I had driven down to Mays Landing near the Jersey Shore to interview her. I had my laptop bag strung over my shoulder and my recorder in my pocket. I felt I looked like a real reporter, but I was a just a student working on her masters project. I wasn't sure what to expect. What if Erin didn't say much? What if I asked the wrong questions? I cracked my knuckles more than once as I walked closer, a nervous habit I could never seem to kick. Knitting magazines adorned the shelf next to her, and a tote with knitting needles and red yarn sat by her feet. She was dressed elegantly with simple ankle- high brown boots that matched her curly long brown hair, jeans, a burgundy corduroy tailored jacket and a gold studded black bracelet. She looked like any other artistic young woman with a hobby. And then I noticed a cane leaning next to her.

"Hi, are you Erin?" I asked.

"Yes, you must be Toni?"

I sat down on the matching chair in front of her so she didn't have to get up. I began rambling about how grateful I was that she had let me interview her and that I had so many questions. I couldn't stop bouncing my knee up and down. I was kind of a mess. This was my first interview for my project on lupus and I was nervous and didn't know how Erin would act. But she instantly put me at ease. She spoke slowly, putting space between each word. It had a soothing effect. Because of her I began to relax. When we got right down to it, she began our interview in the perfect place.

"It's pretty much the tenth anniversary of when I got sick," Erin told me.

She was 35 this year and it was exactly ten years ago at age 25 when she realized life would forever be altered.

Erin Castaldi was born October 19th, 1978. She was the oldest of four and attributes that to her wanting to be a teacher. Erin made money like any other preteen/teenage girl, by babysitting for her neighbors. Erin recalled one child, Jolie, whom she babysat.

"She's a sweetheart. She had Lyme disease. I think. She was a good kid."

Lyme disease wasn't the only thing Jolie had. I had called Jolie a few days before and she explained how lupus affected her life.

"A few years out of high school my hands swelled. They were stiff and hurt and I automatically thought Lyme disease," Jolie said to me over the phone a few days before meeting Erin. "It makes you feel like you're going crazy when doctors can't say what's wrong with you. It was almost a year and the fourth rheumatologist that found I had markers for lupus. With all the symptoms you can find an excuse for them. Tired? I didn't get enough sleep. Hair loss? Too much stress. It took eight to nine months for a diagnosis."

A few years earlier, around the time Erin was 19, similar things started happening to her. They lasted six months.

"I was working in the casinos in Atlantic City. I was a surveillance officer and I worked in the computer room," Erin said. "It started off with one finger was numb. I thought this is so weird. I couldn't bend it. It felt like it was blown up, it was the weirdest oddest thing. I went to see a rheumatologist and my blood work was high for inflammation rate, ANA was high. My SED rate, which measures inflammation, was high. It's based on levels of 300 and I was at 2000 and change. So I started to see a rheumatologist. They prescribed Neurontin and prednisone and that helped. I was out of work for six months with joint pain and other stuff like headaches. I couldn't sit or stand. It hurt. Then I was good. I felt good. I went back to work for about 2 years. I loved it. I was doing great. It was a great job."

With life on the right track Erin would have never imagined the trials that would await her just two years later.

# 2. The Lab

Dear Diary 4-14-11

"Gave two weeks' notice at work. Done in 8 days or so. Dana was surprised and taken aback saying she had big plans for me and that I can stay 1 day a week. I told her I would talk w/ Paul and let her know. Told her because the business is taking off and not because I am sick. They do not know about my illness. I would like to leave the door open for seasonal work." – Erin Castaldi

To Maryat Lee February 11, 1958

"Here I am misinforming my dear friends a mile a minute. No I am not going to Rome nor nowhere else (except Missouri). The doctor as of yesterday says I can't go. You didn't know I had a DREAD DISEASE didja? My father died of the same stuff at the age of 44 but the scientists hope to keep me here until I'm 96 … the name of the dread disease is Lupus Erythematosus, or as we literary people call it, Red Wolf. Anyway, no Europe. I am bearing this with my usual magnificent fortitude." – Flannery O'Connor


**** 

The disease *systemic lupus erythematosus* takes its name from the *Latin* word "*lupus*", meaning *wolf*. The earliest use of the term "lupus" in English literature is in the biography of St. Martin written in the 10th century. During this period, in the Middle Ages, people who had red scars on their faces with lesions and red blotches were thought to have the mark of the wolf – a werewolf to be exact. It was assumed that on a full moon they turned into hideous wolves that stalked their prey.

Today such superstitions have died out. Instead, the medical world has classified all the different types of lupus. Generally lupus is called lupus erythematosus and consists of about four major types: systemic lupus erythematosus, cutaneous lupus, drug-induced lupus, and neonatal lupus. Systemic lupus erythematosus is the most dangerous form of the disease where not only skin is affected but organs, like lung, kidney, heart as well. Cutaneous lupus deals primarily with the skin and includes discoid lupus, in which raised red rashes become thick and scaly usually after being exposed to the sun and may scar. Hair loss may occur at the location of the lesion and may be permanent. Drug-induced lupus typically reverses once the drug is stopped and neonatal lupus, contracted when the mother has lupus, is systemic lupus erythematosus in infants. Most infants can grow out of the disease. Studying mainly systemic lupus erythematosus are scientists from all corners of the immunology field.

****

It was the beginning of the following work week and Uma worked fast on this Monday morning. As usual during the mornings in the lab it was quiet. Quiet as in library quiet. No matter where you walked on the 11th floor, the research floor, you could only hear sounds of a door closing behind you or your shoes squeaking below. Uma was on auto-drive. With her petite delicate hands she worked like a master quickly sucking liquid up into the pipette and depositing it in the small plastic container called an Eppendorf tube. Normally she talked as she worked but not this morning. The only thing on her mind was that for every single day these past two weeks she'd been running experiments on one thing- the paper she submitted to the journal PLOS-ONE a few months ago. Since submitting, the peer reviews of the journal had come back with suggestions on how to make her experiments stronger before they'd publish her work.

She was working with dendritic cells. Dendritic cells are immune cells located all over the body. They activate T and B lymphocytes, which are like weapons factories producing antibodies that fight infection. Uma studied the disease lupus, in which the antibody proteins fight against someone's own organs instead of an invader like a virus. For most people their dendritic cells, B and T lymphocytes work in perfect harmony getting rid of germs that can cause disease, called pathogens, while not attacking the body's own healthy cells. But for others this is not the case. Somewhere along the line, the immune system begins to attack its own cells instead of pathogens and results in what is called "autoimmunity." Autoimmune diseases include ailments such as rheumatoid arthritis, juvenile diabetes and lupus.

I had just started shadowing Uma and her peers who worked under the direction of Dr. Stefania Gallucci. I first became interested in lupus as an undergrad. I studied biology at Ursinus College and the summer going into my senior year I landed an internship with Stefania, a well-respected researcher, in an immunology lab. Immunology is the study of the immune system and Stefania was studying the autoimmune disease systemic lupus erythematosus, whereby dendritic cells tell lymphocytes to make autoantibodies, or antibodies against the body's own tissues. The autoantibodies that are produced can wreak havoc on the victim. Autoantibodies can also cause severe issues with organs such as kidney failure and therefore can be fatal. This is because the autoantibodies bind to the body's cells and molecules, like proteins and DNA, instead of to pathogens and form what are called immune complexes. These immune complexes stick to blood vessel walls. Since there are millions of blood vessels in the kidney it is one organ that is affected. There are also cases like Erin Castaldi, whose central nervous system is affected, leaving her feeling tingly, as if the left side of her body had fallen asleep.

Stefania's research regarding lupus was as exciting as any research I had done as an undergrad. But the lab bench wasn't where I belonged. I liked the people and the atmosphere more than I liked the pipetting and centrifuging. And although I no longer wished to be at the lab bench, I did wish to write about it.

It was now 2013, almost 10 years later. There were some minor changes. I was no longer a pre-medical biology student, but rather in my last year of a masters in writing/journalism program. Stefania had since moved from the University of Pennsylvania, where I had worked, to Temple School of Medicine. I had just driven through Philadelphia north up Broad Street to this new address in order to write an insider's look into her world. North Philadelphia was an area of contrast. In between the dilapidated buildings, multicolored, with slanted shutters and rusting awnings, and overall in bad need of paint, were dorm houses, beautiful lecture halls, or buildings like the building where Stefania worked, a modern-looking research facility called the Medicine Education and Research Building in the Health Science Center. Looking at the facility, I could see why she'd be willing to focus her research in this new spot.

Stefania had told me to get to the lab by 9:20 to make sure I could make the meeting at 9:30. It was 9:20 on the dot when I entered the research building. Perfect. When I had worked for Stefania's lab in the past I had an ID badge and had gotten to know security pretty well. Today, I was a stranger.

"Who are you here to see?" the security guard asked looking down over the tops of her glasses at me.

"Stefania Gallucci, she's a researcher here…"

"Is she expecting you?"

"Yes."

"Do you have her phone number?" The questions continued, especially after Stefania didn't answer the first phone number I gave. Eventually it was sorted out, and relieved, I had an ID tag with a photo and UPC code to boot.

"Temple University Antonia DiBona, 11<sup>th</sup> Floor, Research Department."

I felt official.

I hadn't seen Stefania in close to ten years so I wasn't sure what to expect. The first words that out of my mouth were:

"Do I look any different?"

"No of course not! I mean, do I? Of course not," she said in a thick Italian accent.

Stefania always had a way of being honest about what she thought. Ten years earlier when I interviewed to be an intern she handed me a dry erase marker and told me to come up with a way to test if a certain protein acted as a signal to regulate the expression of another. I had aced every biology/genetics/organic chemistry class I took but never did they ask me to come up with an experiment. To this day I distinctly remember what she said as I stood in front of her desk shell-shocked.

"You want to be a scientist don't you?" she said. "Show me."

I dreamt up an impossibly complicated cocktail of every genetics classroom protocol I could think of. When I was done, I had drawn arrows left to right to diagonal and up and down across the whiteboard in Stefania's office. She concluded it was feasible, unrealistic, but feasible and I think out of the amazing kindness of her heart offered me the internship.

Today it was like no time had passed. Tall, with long brown hair pulled back revealing intense green eyes, she was right again in that she didn't look different.

"What time is it?" Stefania asked.

"9:30"

"Perfect let's get going."

On our way down stairs to the lab meeting we met a young woman carrying books that looked like they weighed on her so heavily she had to brace herself against the elevator door as it was closing. She smiled wide when she saw Stefania.

"Dr. Gallucci do you have a moment to go over what you spoke about in your lecture today? I just have a couple of questions."

She kept smiling.

"Of course, can you come by around 12?"

"Yes. Thank you!"she said.

I've seen this reaction before. It's usually with someone famous. It was like we were in the presence of Sandra Bullock. We stepped out of the elevator leaving the captivated young woman behind. Stefania always walked like she had somewhere important to be and like she was always 10 minutes late. I was working up a small sweat keeping up.

We entered a small conference room with tables set up in rows and a projector at the front. Next to the projector was a man, perhaps in his mid to late twenties, fiddling with his laptop.

"Everyone whisper, make some noise like I'm at the conference," he said.

Paul Gallo, an MD PhD student working for Stefania was preparing his presentation that day for the American College of Rheumatology Annual Meeting in San Diego, held from Oct 25th-30th 2013.

"I hope they stay on time at the meeting. It's a national conference so I'm sure they don't mess around," he said as he kept fidgeting.

On the screen in big bold print read "Bacterial Amyloids Promote Type I Interferon Production and Accelerate Autoimmunity." One of the many large scope goals of Stefania's lab is to pinpoint causes of autoimmunity, or why the body's immune system starts attacking its own organs. In conjunction with Cagal Tukel's lab, they tested Curli, a protein component secreted by

*Enterobacteriaceae,* a type of bacteria that live in our gut. Slide after slide tried to prove their

hypothesis that Curli can cause autoimmunity. Many researchers have hinted that outside

bacterial infection can initiate lupus, but Stefania's lab wanted to show proof. The first slide

showed *in vitro* studies where Curli caused cytokine production in bone marrow dendritic cells

of mice. Why is that relevant? Cytokines are proteins like interleukin-6 (IL-6) and interleukin-12

(IL-12) and can cause inflammation. Inflammation is a major problem in patients with lupus and

Paul showed that Curli stimulates the immune cells to produce these cytokines. To further

ground their proof that Curli cause autoimmunity like lupus, they studied it in vivo, meaning

inside the mouse. The last slide showed that when mice were injected with Curli there were

higher levels of autoantibodies in the blood. Autoantibodies produced by the human or mouse B-

cells attack the body's own DNA instead of foreign matter. It's a classic sign of lupus. Anti-

DNA autoantibodies (Or ANA) in a patient's blood are one of the signals to doctors that the

patient has the disease.

The presentation finished at eight minutes forty- seven seconds. The suggestions and

corrections to the presentation lasted twice as long and were grueling.

"I need you to say more things," Stefania said. "Let's go back to the first slide. That

picture? Get rid of it. It's too complicated and doesn't say anything."

Paul typed a reminder to himself.

Second slide

"Start with the biofilm and say how it has the amyloid in it."

Next slide.

"The stain should be on a black background," someone said.

"Say WE DISCOVERED, not 'it seems to say.' You need to be proud of our discovery," Stefania added

The suggestions from all 7 people in the room continued for all 14 slides.

"Change the graphs from a line graph to a bar graph; it's easier to read."

"Change the labels of the bar graph from diagonal to vertical."

"Don't forget to add a slide thanking everyone."

"Change the title so IL-6 and IL-12 are prominent."

Paul took everything in stride, simply nodding and typing each suggestion to remember it later.

One particular aspect of his talk struck my curiosity. He said something about the mice not showing signs of the disease and was keeping his fingers crossed they did. I asked him what he meant.

"Normally in mice with full onset of lupus, proteins will start to show in the urine indicating kidney damage," he said. "Kidneys are tricky though because most of the kidney must be damaged before proteins start to show in the urine. As of yet, none of the mice from these experiments showed proteins in their urine."

"Is that bad?" I asked.

"Well honestly we don't know if it's bad or good. It's an unexpected result."

"What will you do now?'

"We will continue to monitor the urine. And then we have to figure out why they are not showing signs of lupus."

And so the research continues, the fight to finding a cure never-ending.

# 3. The Literary Side

Dear Diary, 3-3-08

It seems as if I need to be drug to the ER. This chest pain seems to be the sharpest and most stubborn I have yet encountered. I can't seem to get comfortable w/ the notion of my being ill and all that goes w/ it. It makes me do all of which I dread. Be stagnant, explain myself constantly, feel useless, when on the brink of good health I feel like I am getting [pushed toward the edge of a] precipice. I have no control. I have no say and the unpredictability of my fall makes it all the more frustrating and humbling. – Erin Castaldi

To Sister Marielle Gable, July 5, 1964

"The wolf, I'm afraid, is inside tearing up the place. I've been in the hospital 50 days already this year. At present I'm just home from the hospital and have to stay in bed. I have an electric typewriter and I write a little every day but I'm not allowed to do much. I'll count on your prayers." – Flannery O'Connor


***


There is no cure. To this day, dating back centuries, those four words stood for the prognosis of lupus. It is like a beast inside, ravaging the organs, central nervous system, joints, or skin. If lupus affects the skin, most times it shows as a "butterfly rash" because it looks like the shape of a butterfly. The red, scaly rash also resembles something a bit more sinister, the bite of a wolf.

When Flannery O'Connor wrote to her friend Sister Marielle Gable on July 5th 1964 about the "wolf", it was one month before she died.

She was a story teller by heart. Once she wrote the story of a girl with an artificial leg who had to go back to her country home after earning her Ph.D. and live with a mother who could not appreciate her degree.

"The girl had taken the Ph.D. in philosophy and this left Mrs. Hopewell at a complete loss," the story goes. "You could say, 'My daughter is a nurse,' or 'My daughter is a schoolteacher,' or even, 'My daughter is a chemical engineer.' You could not say, 'My daughter is a philosopher.' That was something that ended with the Greeks and Romans."

She wrote of a girl that belonged in academia but had to live at her homestead on a farm. She wrote of a girl that not only had a bum leg but a weak heart and wasn't supposed live past 45.

"Joy had made it plain that if it had not been for this condition, she would be far from these red hills and good country people," says the narrator of the story. "She would be in a university lecturing to people who knew what she was talking about."

The character, Joy, changed her name to Helga which she considered an ugly name. Helga held her current life in disdain. She couldn't live the life she wanted and in the end of the story she was left alone, her leg stolen, and totally dependent on her mother, completely opposite of the self-sufficient woman she wished to be.

Did the author, Flannery O'Connor relate? Most likely, yes. Her short stories show the bitter truth to the reality of life. Flannery O'Connor died at age 39 in 1964 due to complications of lupus.

Over Christmas, as usual, I asked for a variety of books, but I wanted one in particular, Flannery O'Connor's *The Complete Stories*. It won the National Book Award for Fiction in

1972, eight years after her death. When I first learned she had lupus I was intrigued and dug deeper. Flannery O'Connor made her living as a novelist and short story writer. After her Bachelor's degree in Social Sciences from Georgia State College for Women she was accepted into the prestigious Iowa's Writer's Workshop, and I was further interested to find she studied journalism, like me. After she was diagnosed with lupus in 1951, she had to move home to the family farm in Milledgeville, Georgia.

As I read *The Complete Stories,* one story that caught my eye was titled "Revelation." I googled it and found it was the last story she wrote before she died.

Flannery O'Connor's last short story goes something like this. Mrs. Turpin considered herself righteous and good, but in reality was judgmental and a racist. It took a girl who she thought was ugly to throw a book at her and hit her square above the eye to change her view. And then the girl said, "Go back to hell where you came from, you old wart hog." That threw a wrench into everything Mrs. Turpin thought about herself. She cried out to her Lord, "How am I hog and me, both? How am I saved and from hell too?" "Why me? she rumbled. "It's no trash around here, black or white, that I haven't given to. And break my neck to the bone every day working. And do for the church." Then Mrs. Turpin saw a vision of every different sort of people including her sort. They were dignified, "yet, she could see by their shock and altered faces that even their virtues were being burned away." Mrs. Turpin saw a vision of "her" people bringing up the rear of the procession into heaven that she imagined against the backdrop of a setting sun. "Her" people were behind all those she considered less than herself.

Flannery O'Connor had to have contemplated death quite a lot, considering her bouts with lupus flares and the struggle against medicine complications. I think it is because of her illness she decided to write a story like "Revelation." It was as if her disease only cemented a desire to write about what really matters. She knew her time was limited and this last story shows a desire to write about something bigger thing than herself. She wrote a commentary on morality. Her struggle with lupus can also be seen in her earlier stories with characters like Joy of "Good Country People." Scholars of Flannery O'Connor's work have said that her main characters normally have some flaw, much like Joy's prosthetic leg. The leg could very well be a metaphor for Flannery O'Connor's own struggles with lupus. Flannery O'Connor was one famous writer with lupus, but lupus attacks everyone, famous or not, without mercy. Lupus is a hidden disease, but its effects are most felt by the patient. Erin was no different.

# 4. When Things Went Wrong

Dear Diary 10-11-05

"I am lying here in the hospital bed. The only thing I look forward to in the day is my pain shot. 2 mg of dilaudid every 4 hours. It makes the pain a little better than bearable. If I could really manage my pain well and consistently I could resume some sort of life and independence. Even if that means a slight intoxication or heavy drug. I just want to be as pain free as possible. I cannot live w/ it so constantly for much longer." – Erin Castaldi

To Louise and Tom Gossett May 12, 1964

"Well our state has changed considerably since you last heard from me. I have been in the hospital again and now am in bed full time. That operation started up the old trouble and I am back on the cortisone and doing none too well- though I feel no pain, only weakness. Yesterday I had a blood transfusion ... so today I got the energy to write some letters." – Flannery O'Connor

\*\*\*\*

It was March 2003. Erin had decided to become a paramedic. She had enrolled in Camden County College's Associates Program in Paramedic Sciences, the only one of its kind. At age 25 she was already recently divorced and living the single life in Waretown, New Jersey near the Jersey shore. She commuted about a half hour to work as an EMT in Whiting, New Jersey, and commuted over an hour to attend classes in Cherry Hill and Blackwood. She shared the house with two other girls and the rent was cheap, 400 bucks a month. It was awesome. She was awesome. She was motivated and active and a young girl with a promising future.

One night after coming home from work as an EMT she drove to her boyfriend's place.

She was still in her brown pants, black rubber soled shoes and white collared uniform when she strolled in. The two of them began a night together as usual. Beer, wings and cards. At the time Erin was only taking Neurontin to dull her nerves for the finger problem she contracted a few years earlier. She thought perhaps that was the reason that after just one beer she felt drunk, really drunk. As if that wasn't embarrassing enough, her boyfriend had to carry her upstairs to bed.

The next morning Erin turned over in bed and let out a small groan. *What happened?* She winced at each pulse of the blood vessels in her temples. From the joints in her hand down to her feet everything ached something awful. Although it was a gray winter day the light from the window was blinding. She felt like she had drunk half a case of beer the night before. She decided not to drive back to her place, but directly to her parents' house instead. The whole side of her body, including her legs, was numb. She crawled up the stairs in her parents' house to her old room. Erin took the covers and pulled them up over her head. The pins and needles of her left side would not go away. She tried to sleep but she couldn't. Her parents made the decision to bring her to the hospital.

It had been one week and she was still in the ICU. Her fever reached 104 degrees Fahrenheit and would not come down. Test after test was performed. What did she have? At some point the diagnoses ranged from multiple sclerosis to Lyme disease. It took six years after Erin's first bouts with numbness in her hand, but the doctors finally pinned down her diagnosis. Erin was suffering from a lupus flare. Her whole body was ignited with pain, redness, and swelling. Her immune system's cells were causing her body to be inflamed.

Cells are the basic unit of life. They make up all living things and have different roles. Those involved with lupus are the white blood cells like T and B lymphocytes and originate in the bone marrow or the tissue inside our bones. Dendritic cells then "talk" to T lymphocytes,

which then "talk" to B lymphocytes which create antibodies to kill what they consider dangerous

invaders.

****

Dendritic cells are partly activated through their TLRs, toll-like receptors. TLR-7 and

TLR-9 have been implicated in the disease. They are proteins that traverse the dendritic cell

membrane and recognize the DNA or RNA sequence of pathogens like viruses. They then cause

an immune response with inflammation. It is this inflammation that causes the excruciating pain

that many sufferers of lupus feel.

A few months ago, Uma submitted a manuscript showing a significant result. A certain

protein suppresses the effects of these TLRs. If the TLRs could be suppressed then maybe they

could find a way to stop the onset of lupus. At lunch Uma explained the process of getting

published while inhaling her food in the 20 minutes she had between experiments.

"First you submit the manuscript with your results," she said in between bites. "Then the

reviewers for the journal find areas that can be improved upon and things that need further

testing. Then you have a few months to make the changes and resubmit." She sighed. "You *hope*

they will publish your latest findings."

"I'm super stressed out this week," she said, although you could never tell in the lab. She

was meticulous and deliberate with everything she did. She worked quickly but it never seemed

rushed. She just made it look easy.

"What are you doing now?" I asked at the lab bench after lunch, as I saw her pour

something that looked like milk onto blotting paper.

"It IS milk. Actually it's milk proteins. I pour it on here to stop nonspecific binding,"she said.

Uma was performing a western blot -- a standard in cell biology. She was trying to see if TLR-9 showed up in her dendritic cell sample. Because TLR-9 is a type of protein there is an antibody available that binds ONLY to it. Uma first treated the blotting paper with the dendritic cell sample with milk proteins, or albumin, to make sure the first antibody she added did not just bind randomly to the blotting paper. This first antibody binds to the TLR9. Then a second antibody is added to bind to the first antibody. The second antibody is fluorescent, so if Uma detects a color she knows the TLR9 is present.

She swirled the blotting paper in the milk proteins with eyes focused on her technique.

"It's a two day process," Uma said not looking up. "On the first day you put the primary antibody and let it sit overnight. Then the next day you put the secondary antibody and see if you detect color, or if there is protein present."

I saw Uma later that day. I wasn't too keen on taking home a 600 dollar book Stefania lent me so I was in the break area making copies when Uma came in and plopped down on the couch behind me.

"Did you find the protein you were looking for?" I asked.

"No … not yet," she said.

"Isn't that bad?" I asked.

"That's the way it is in science. You don't always get your hypothesis," she said. "But that's ok, I still have more tests. We will see what happens."

Like everyone in Stefania's lab Uma exhibited an extraordinary amount of patience. When it comes to science you have to expect unexpected results. I remember as an intern if I didn't get the result I wanted I damn near had a heart attack. I looked/acted anxious more days than not, while Uma continued work as usual. That part of her hadn't changed.

Later that week I emailed her asking about her results. I received an email from her a few days later at 4:36 am. It said:

"As you know the experiments do not work straightforward. Needs a lot of standardization and testing of various conditions. Finally after two weeks of hectic work I think I have some data that I can show as mechanism. Hopefully the reviewers are OK with our revision and accept our paper for publication!!!"

# 5. The Gallucci/Caricchio Force

Dear Diary, 8/19/10

"I feel like a weirdo all the time – especially in the summer. I have to be a homebody because everyone I know hears how bad the sun is for me. It's so disappointing. The sun is not that bad w/ clothes and sunscreen I don't know if it is really detrimental. I wish the sun were not my enemy." – Erin Castaldi

To Cecil Dawkins, March 6, 1959

"The sun is greatly restricting my activities right now and will continue to do so, I'm afraid. The doctor says I can't go out of the house without stockings, gloves, long sleeves and large hat. The spectacle of me in this get-up all summer is depressing to my imagination. We are having green glass put in the car … Well cheers." – Flannery O'Connor


\*\*\*\*

It was 1999 – the year of the third installment of Harry Potter – Harry Potter and the Prisoner of Azkaban. It was the year everyone caught the Y2K bug and hoarded bottles of water in their basement for the moment the clocks switched over. It was pre-9/11 back when everyone in your party could accompany you to the gate. One such traveler had arrived from Italy three years before and decided not to go back. From what was supposed to be her one year fellowship experience abroad, she extended her stay indefinitely. Dr. Stefania Gallucci came to the United States to finish her fellowship at The National Institute of Health (NIH), a part of the U.S. Department of Health and Human Services, and one of the world's foremost medical research centers. After one year she was offered a post-doc at the same lab to continue her studies. She accepted and never went back to Italy. At the time, she never thought her research would open her up to the nebulous and fascinating world of lupus.

Ever since she was three years old Stefania wanted to be a doctor. She didn't care what kind of doctor it was; she knew she wanted to wear the lab coat and to help others. At one point she wanted to be a cardiologist, and then a psychiatrist and then a family doctor. Whenever she went for a visit she would watch the doctors fascinated by everything they did. In a town that wasn't a city but wasn't exactly rural either, she grew up 30 miles south of Rome in the late 80s. In high school she narrowed her focus and decided she wanted to do clinical research, so when she applied and was accepted to medical school in Rome, her internship experiences all involved clinical pathology research in a lab. Her first internship experience was in an immunology lab and the seed was planted. Many years later, as I sat in Stefania's office with the recorder clicked on and a pen and paper in my hand, I asked Stefania why she chose lupus research. She explained that sometimes in life it is the choices you make that meet with opportunities given. She was given the opportunity to work in an immunology lab but chose to continue the research in the United States for her post-doc.

"I was interested in autoimmunity because that was the first lab I was in," she said. "But in Italy I recognized I wanted more basic training. The NIH offered more basic research with dendritic cells. This is where I wanted to focus."

One day I googled Stefania Gallucci's name out of curiosity. Among headshots at Temple University one image stood out from the rest. It was of the Fellows Award for Research Excellence competition at the NIH in 1999. There, standing next to a poster board that read in big bold letters, "Death, Danger and Dendritic Cells," was a young version of the woman in whose office I now sat at Temple University some 15 years later. A wild mane of wavy hair was pulled back by glasses resting on the top of her head. Her eyes were focused on the gentleman speaking to her as if she digested every word he said. It's no surprise she was honored for her work with dendritic cells that year.

In 1999 Stefania stumbled onto something quite novel. She had been studying bone marrow derived dendritic cells. I like to imagine dendritic cells like the hall monitors of your elementary school. They scout the halls of your body for invaders that do not belong. They are also like messy eaters because they ingest the invader and leave some crumbs on their face. These crumbs, or fragments of the foreign invader are displayed on the dendritic cell surface and just like generals in a war they direct the T and B lymphocytes to produce antibodies to kill the invader.

Stefania took a deceased mouse, as she had done thousands of times before, and removed muscle tissue from the femur and the tibia. She cut both ends of the bone with scissors and then flushed out the bone marrow using a syringe. Stefania was used to this procedure. The push and the pull of the syringe almost had a rhythm to it. The dendritic cells (DCs) were placed in wells and incubated in a red tinted special medium that kept the cells alive.

"Danger, Death and Dendritic Cells." Death. It is an unfriendly word, but at the same time a necessary one. All living things must die. Cells are no different. Cell death can belong to one of two classes- apoptotic and necrotic. Apoptotic cell death is like when leaves fall off trees in the autumn. It is pre-planned, pre-programmed death so that new cells can replace old ones. It is not damaging. Necrotic death is like cell murder. When a cell is stressed either through a toxin or trauma or infection it is destroyed from the inside out. It explodes inside the body, releasing its contents. Necrosis can be devastating, causing disaster like gangrene, which is the build-up of dead, murdered cells. Stefania was interested in necrosis.

"Danger Death and Dendritic Cells." She treated some DCs with the insides of the dead necrotic cells. Unlike anything seen before the DCs became activated. She stared at computer image of the fluorescent markers. The data looked like mounds of ants, each dot being a marker that showed the DCs were activated. The computer printout showed a clear dense mound of dots when the DCs were treated with necrotic cell debris. The results showed that danger signals from necrotic cells can activate dendritic cells. Up until this point immunologists thought DCs were only activated by foreign invaders. Now, for the first time, Stefania and her lab showed they could be activated from the body's own dying cells. The necrotic cells released "danger signals" which signaled the DCs to be activated and start the immune response.

"Before our paper, immunologists believed the immune system and dendritic cells are only activated by infection. We were the first to show that is not the case," Stefania explained to me in her interview. "We opened the new field of research about endogenous danger signals that are molecules normally hidden from the immune system that are released by cells that are stressed or dying by necrotic death."

In other words, the dendritic cells do not have to be activated directly by foreign pathogens; they can be activated by cells inside the body that died by necrosis.

A few years later, in 2001, when Stefania moved to a position as an assistant professor at University of Pennsylvania, she had been talking about lupus with her husband Dr. Roberto Caricchio, the same future husband she had met in high school, and who was a researcher in rheumatology. It was like a double shot of scientific brainpower. Two experts in the field literally worked day and night as they exchanged scientific ideas. Roberto was studying lupus, and they discussed the disease almost every night. Fifteen years later and they still have the same passion and drive to win the fight against this harsh disease.

"So before having children we used to talk about science all the time. We used to plan experiments at home. Since we have children, the children attract most of our attention because when we stay with them it's their time. Most of the time is spent with them. But we have discussions also at home," Stefania said. "There are times when, especially the oldest, Tiberio, asks a question about our research and we talk about lupus together as a family."

When Stefania joined University of Pennsylvania and Children's Hospital of Philadelphia in 2001 there were quite a few labs focused solely on lupus. At that point Stefania now had the basic research background from the NIH and she brought her expertise in dendritic cells to the world of lupus at Penn. So began the world of dendritic cells in the context of lupus. Today her office at Temple is on the same floor as her husband's. Both study lupus. Dr. Caricchio is a researcher, but a medical doctor as well, and so is concerned about lupus in human patients as well as in mice. One day I caught him in the hallway, well, caught isn't really the word. I had set up shop at a table in the hallway two doors down from him and waited. It worked. When I "ran into him," he offered me an inside look into his world, I accepted.

****

They seemed to speak in code.

"C3 and C4 complement is down."

"ESR is up."

"CRP is up."

Some of it I understood,

"Is WBC down?"

"What about RBC?"

I thought that must mean white blood cell count and red blood cell count and for a moment I liked to imagine I had understood the rest.

I had arrived at 3322 N. Broad Street with my notebook and pen, laptop, and winter coat. When I entered the hospital, they directed me past the patients in the waiting room and through a locked door to the main part of the hospital. Around the corner to my left was a little room with men and women in white lab coats with stethoscopes around their necks. Some were seated in front of computers with tables of information. I sat down in the corner without taking off my coat because there was no place to put it and quickly realized I didn't need my laptop. Doctors came in and out of the tiny room lightning fast. There would be no place for sit down interviews here.

Temple University Hospital was just a block down from the research center where scientist Stefania Gallucci's team worked on lupus at the cellular level. Here at the hospital a different kind of doctor attacked lupus. It was a battlefield, and MDs like Dr. Roberto Caricchio, Dr. Philip Cohen, and Dr. Steven Burney were the generals training MD fellows out in the field and treating patient after patient who showed signs of lupus.

Like his wife Dr. Roberto Caricchio packed quite a punch in the fight against lupus. Roberto was a researcher and a clinician. He had invited me to follow along with him on Tuesday mornings, when he mainly saw his lupus patients.

Dr. Caricchio was a slim man, tall and thin. Must be because he walked just as fast if not faster than his wife. He wore rimless glasses, had light brown hair that thinned a bit at the top, and wore a white colored shirt and black dress pants. When I met him that Tuesday his navy blue tie peeked through behind his white lab coat.

There was no time for long introductions. One second after I said hi, an Indian woman, a fellow, also donning a white lab coat, started talking to Dr. Caricchio. A fellow is usually a doctor who has finished his/her residency and wants to undergo a period of continuing medical training.

"I have *nine* patients today," she sounded exasperated.

"It's ok. You won't die," Dr. Caricchio smiled. "Tell me about your patient."

"She is a 25 year old woman. She was diagnosed with lupus in February 2008 with reactive lymphadenopathy. Biopsy ruled out infection and malignancy. Polyarthritis of the small joints, Raynaud's disease, oral ulcers, recurrent exudative pleural effusion. Leukopenia. She was on Imuran."

Dr. Caricchio and his student continued to speak in such language with Dr. Caricchio answering her questions with questions.

"And that symptom would be secondary to what?" he asked.

"Well she has swollen glands," the fellow responded.

'Is it painful?" Dr. Caricchio asked.

"No, I mean I don't think so," she responded.

"Did you ask?" Dr. Caricchio asked.

"No," she said.

"What does it mean if it's painful? It means inflammation." Dr. Caricchio answered his own question this time.

"Let's go talk to the patient. Let's go see. Toni, do you want to come? "

Up until this point I had been oblivious, just scribbling down everything I could catch and try and make sense of it.

"Oh, I can come with you? "

"Yes, yes. But you need a lab coat. Get a lab coat upstairs."

Dr. Caricchio and his student headed toward the patient, while I went in search of a lab coat.

I found a hanger for my winter coat because I had worked up quite a sweat downstairs. Finding a lab coat proved a bit trickier. I stopped a secretary in the hallway and told her my predicament. Bless her heart, she stopped and found me a coat of a previous student. It was a little small, but mostly I looked the part. She wrote my name on a sticky label and taped it over the former student's name.

It was odd. I walked downstairs past patients waiting in the hallway and they all looked up to me with new interest. I could feel their stares as I tried to find refuge in the little doctors meeting room away from their gaze.

A different student was talking to Dr. Caricchio now.

"She is a 52 year old African American. Her major complaint is fatigue," said the fellow. Dr. Caricchio nodded, "Okay."

"She is super healthy though. She's on an all anti-oxidant diet," the fellow stressed the last part.

Dr. Caricchio didn't seem fazed.

"Oh fine, good." As if to say, oh yeah sure the anti-oxidant diet will cure it.

"She wants to try alternative medicine," said the fellow.

"Ok, but let's see what we can do first," Dr. Caricchio said.

I followed Dr. Caricchio and his fellow to Exam Room 6. Dr. Caricchio never missed a beat. He listened to the patient, stared her straight in the eyes, nodded and without the slightest hesitation responded in the most logical manner.

"I'm so tired all the time," the patient said.

"Fatigue is a symptom of lupus. What have you been up to?

"I'm a Certified Nursing Assistant. I'm trying to get my LPN license."

"Stress can cause lupus flares. Let's do some blood work and see if it's really a flare. I also want a chest X ray just to get a base line. Maybe let's try prednisone. Buy ourselves some time."

Dr. Caricchio left the patient with the fellow and walked back past the nurses' station to the room with all the doctors. The doctors seemed to have no interaction with anyone else except the patients and themselves.

The young female fellow was waiting. She wanted to talk to Dr. Caricchio about another patient. It was only 10:00 in the morning and I felt as if we had seen half the patients in the waiting area. Dr. Caricchio, however, was not fazed. His funny, light-hearted sensibility hadn't gone anywhere.

"She was diagnosed in 1994,"the female fellow said.

"Don't believe it," Dr. Caricchio said,

"She was diagnosed at Einstein Medical," she said.

"Even worse," said Dr. Caricchio.

He obviously wasn't being serious, but I marveled at his energy to crack jokes when I was in bad need of a nap.

I followed him around the rest of the morning. I heard him warn patients to stop everything from smoking cigarettes to smoking cocaine.

"Ay ménage! You really have to stop that," he'd say with that little Italian phrase sneaking in when he was really passionate.

When I followed Dr. Caricchio and a fellow in to see one patient, an African American woman in her fifties, I saw red blotches all across her skin.

"It itches so bad. It feels like a burn," she said.

The young Indian male fellow made an observation that it didn't look like cellulitis.

"It's not diffuse. It's localized," he said.

Dr. Caricchio explained to the patient that he meant it's not everywhere; it's just in certain spots.

"They look like insect bites to me," Dr. Caricchio said.

"No, they're not insect bites. Mmm mmm. No not insect bites. The dermatologist told me it's lupus." She stared straight at Dr. Caricchio, indignant.

"Discoid lupus doesn't come and go. It comes and stays and modifies the skin and goes. And the blotches are warm, like bites. I don't think it's worth a biopsy. We can put cream. Hydrocortisone. Call us in a few weeks to say if the medicine helped or not."

Back in the doctor's meeting area Dr. Caricchio discussed the patient with Dr. Berney, his senior. Sometimes patients with lupus show rashes on their skin when they are exposed to the sun. They did not believe this was such the case.

They wanted to send her to Dr. Gil Yosipovitch, an expert in the itch, and their talks continued from there. I only stayed another hour, but it was clear that one by one they battled lupus and its effects in every patient they saw. Lupus affects every patient differently. It was most severe in Erin's case.

# 6. Tibetan Lion on Flowers

Dear Diary 9-22-05

"I hate life. I don't have faith in anything. I've tried Buddhism and it gave me peace, but only reinforces what I want to do with my life. Help others. I wanted to be a powerfully positive presence in the lives of those I'm near and I can't. I'm always in pain and I feel myself falling down more often. It's getting harder to pick myself back up. I try so hard to have faith in myself and I cannot. Life has no meaning. How can I heal my mind when my body is all I can focus on? It's just one long series of day time TV, nighttime sitcoms, and family drama … Perhaps in the next life, the dreams and goals of this one unfulfilled will guide me in the future." – Erin Castaldi

To Elizabeth Fenwick Way April 1956

"When you feel better, having the right medicine in you, the emotional situation will be less of a strain. Everybody now talks about it's all-in-the-mind. When I was in the hospital even the nurse's aides that didn't have sense enough to do anything but empty the ice-water were full of that chatter" – Flannery O'Connor

****

Back in 2003 and after two weeks at the hospital, with a clear diagnosis of systemic lupus erythematosus, Erin heard the words "discharged." Having been pumped full of steroids and immunosuppressive drugs, she would not be going home to her beloved roommates and the freedom it offered. She would have to go back home to her parents' house. Erin's mom helped her daughter hobble up the stairs to the guest room that had once been her bedroom.

It was six months later. On one of those perfect summer days, a day when Erin would have worn a sun dress, when the temperature was in the 80s and there was a warm breeze, Erin heard the back door open and shut. Her family, her mom and dad and brothers and sisters were

downstairs on the back porch. All Erin could do was look out the window and remember what it

was like to walk on her own. She couldn't do much of anything alone anymore. She couldn't

walk or go to the bathroom alone. In her eyes she was a failure. She went from being an athletic

ambitious driven woman to this girl in bed in her parents' house on tons of medications and in

horrendous pain just 24/7. She went from being a woman living a full life -- one who was

recently divorced and learning to live the single life, to being completely devastated by disease.

For a full year Erin saw only the lavender walls and white wicker furniture of her old

bedroom. For one whole year Erin left the bedroom only to go to the bathroom. The time spent

was marked by which TV show was airing. Queer Eye for the Straight Guy, Maury and reruns of

Friends were her favorite. She would pass the time by writing in her journal and reading.

Eventually a year passed and she did get better, but she was never really the same.

Erin can't hold a job, she told me. I couldn't help but feel bad about my opening

conversation back at the coffee shop when Erin asked me to talk about myself. I was a public

school teacher, I travelled and had lived in Europe, I now was a grad student and I interned at a

publisher. The last job Erin had was almost three years ago. Before she turned 25 she had plans

of joining the Peace Corps and working abroad. Now she had a different job-like routine. It starts

with applying a pain patch, fentanyl, every three days. Then it's two different types of pain

management pills, taken as needed. She takes about four pills in the morning, three in the

afternoon, and five at night. Twelve pills a day.

I had traveled halfway to the Jersey shore, to the coffee shop, to listen to Erin that night. I

was there to tell her story. Sitting across from her, I noticed there was a tattoo on her right arm.

"What is that a tattoo of?" I asked.

"Oh, it's a Tibetan lion on flowers. It's supposed to bring cheerfulness and positivity. I need to remember to be positive. I can be a little negative sometimes."

Listening to Erin talk, I thought the opposite. Of course, it was easy to be negative when at age 25 she was bed ridden for a year and then could only transport herself by wheelchair and then walker. Of course, it was easy to be negative when on a good day she still needed to use a cane. Quite the contrary, she seemed extremely positive in such circumstances. Her answers to my questions were anything but sad.

"I try and concentrate on what having this disease allows me to do and that it allows me to be the teacher I always wanted to be," Erin said. "I teach ESL to adults and that's amazing and I help people improve themselves in this country and that's great. That's pretty awesome. I do creative stuff. I knit, I paint, I draw," Erin said.

I was quite taken by the young woman sitting across from me. I wasn't sure if I could embrace life as she had given her circumstances. It didn't seem fair.

"What is the most difficult aspect of the disease?" I asked.

"What's difficult is I don't look sick," she said. "It's really hard for people to understand it's an inside disease and you're not going to see it on the outside except for the rash that you can cover with makeup and the cane, you can't tell I'm sick." It was true, now that she pointed it out there was a slight reddish tone on her cheeks covered by foundation. Her face was round and puffy, a side effect from the steroids, but was framed nicely by the wave of her hair. She joked about that too. Apparently the medication had given her naturally straight hair a lot of curl.

"I always wanted curly hair. Benefit of the steroids I guess," she said.

"When you first got sick did you talk to others about the disease?" I asked.

"No, I didn't talk to people about it. Nobody but my inner circle knew. There's just so much to the disease I didn't want to tell people."

From personal experience I had learned Erin was right. Whenever I mentioned lupus, most people had some vague idea ranging from thinking it was muscular problems to thinking it was a form of cancer. It's easy to confuse lupus with cancer. Severe cases of lupus are treated with drugs that suppress the immune system, like some used in chemotherapy, because patients with lupus have a malfunctioning immune system. Lupus mainly affects women of child bearing age (15-44) however ten percent of individuals diagnosed with the disease are men. About 1.5 million Americans suffer from lupus and women of color are two to three times more likely to develop the disease. Erin, being Caucasian, was an exception. The disease seemed to have grabbed hold of her and would not let go. But Erin would learn to fight back.

# 7. Her Adventurous Side

Dear Diary 10-23-05

"My NYC excursion is over and now time to get back to real life. 2 doc appts. Tomorrow. Went to Chinatown today. Was wheeled through the streets in a wheel chair. Hurt my pride but it was worth the hit to my ego. I would never have been able to walk around so much had I not had help of moving." – Erin Castaldi

[1]To "A"[1] November 10, 1955

"I have decided I must be a pretty pathetic sight with these crutches. I was in Atlanta the other day in Davidson's. An old lady got on the elevator behind me and as soon as I turned around she fixed me with a moist gleaming eye and said in a loud voice, 'Bless you, darling!' I felt exactly like the Misfit and I gave her a weakly lethal look, whereupon greatly encouraged, she grabbed my arm and whispered (very loud) in my ear. 'Remember what they said to John at the gate, darling!' It was not my floor but I got off and I suppose the old lady was astounded at how quick I could get away on crutches. I have a one-legged friend and I asked her what they said to John at the gate. She said she reckoned they said, 'The lame shall enter first.' This may be because the lame will be able to knock everybody else aside with their crutches." – Flannery O'Connor

\*\*\*\*

I stared at my phone. I picked it up and searched the contacts for "Erin Castaldi." My finger hovered over the "call" button. I didn't want to call again but it had been a couple of

---

[1] In the book *The Habit of Being* of Flannery O'Connor's personal letters "A" was a friend that wanted to remain anonymous.

weeks and Erin hadn't called me back and declined to hang out. My mind raced through different possibilities from her being in a wheelchair to being in bed doubled over in pain. I was worried. Later that week the phone rang and I rushed to answer it.

"How are you? Is everything ok?" were the first words out of my mouth.

She explained that she tripped on some ice and sprained her right ankle. She had to use her cane to walk, which inflamed her chest cavity once more. She couldn't help but laugh at herself and then said that the last couple of days she had been feeling much better. I let out a nervous laugh, oh sure tripped on some ice how funny, and heaved out a sigh. Erin had become more to me than just a subject for my story. We had met a few times without the usual journalist/interviewee scenario – just us hanging out. She picked the best activities, like the first time we met up at "Arts on Asbury" a small Art Gallery in Ocean City, New Jersey.

"Isn't it neat?" Erin asked me when I entered the gallery not much bigger than a living room, but with paintings covering every square inch from the floor to the ceiling. Erin looked like she belonged with a scarf she knitted and beautiful green beaded jewelry she made herself. Actually she did belong to the Ocean City Fine Arts League. And it was neat.

Another time Erin and I met for lunch at the Mays Landing Diner. We sat in quintessential vinyl booth with paper place mats littered with local business listings. She pulled out a sketchbook.

"I took a drawing foundation course three or four years ago through continuing- ed through high school. She taught foundations like dimension and distance," Erin said. "I had never been able to draw- just stick figures. I always wanted to be creative."

I took one art class when I was 28 to spend some time with my grandfather who loved oil painting. Being a perfectionist in school I had never felt like the student who needed extra help until I tried to draw a wooden 3-D model on a 2-D piece of paper. Madness. So when I saw Erin's work I was impressed.

Erin's creativity spilled over into her personal life as well. When she called me Saturday morning, she wanted to discuss her upcoming big plans.

"I guess it was my idea," Erin said.

About a year ago, one day Erin was remembering the life plans she had for herself before she got sick. She had always loved to travel, wanted to work for the Peace Corps actually, and now for the past ten years she'd been mostly in New Jersey. She stared out of the window in her rented home. Things started to dawn on her. She had no real ties to an area; they didn't even own this house. She had no kids either. What was stopping her from making a change in her life? Lupus?

"Ha!" she thought. "I'm not afraid of you."

That night she dropped some hints to her husband Paul, the same Paul she divorced in 2002 and then remarried in 2007. Finally, she asked about living abroad. Paul hated to fly so the idea didn't excite him as much as it did her.

"Cross country road trip!" they said.

That stuck. Now, only three months from their goal Erin was chatting all about it over the phone.

"The cross country road trip idea started when my dad was diagnosed with Parkinson's and it was a really an uncertain time," Erin said. "My dad went from never needing aspirin at 59 to all of a sudden having a progressively degenerative disease. He takes seven different meds at six different times. I kind of freaked out and went a little crazy. I thought, already having a chronic illness, I understand the importance of making every day the best you can, whether doing what you want or helping others or being creative, but when my dad was diagnosed it's like I have to do something. *I can't just be another sick person who is just sick and at home and my husband works.  I didn't plan on having a mediocre life before I got sick and I didn't want one after."*

# 8. The LFA

Dear Diary 6-20-06

"I attended my 1st official board meeting w/ the Lupus Foundation of America of South

Jersey. Meeting was called to order, minutes were taken down and I got to vote on more than one

foundation issue. They see me as a person w/opinions, ideas, experience; not as someone sick

and unable to care for herself. It is so refreshing. It was breathtakingly exhilarating. I felt

appreciated, inspired, spiritually renewed and have been having the best few days my body has

had since my illness began."—Erin Castaldi

****

Stefania and her hundreds of colleagues all battling Erin's disease are, in a way, the

support team rooting for her on her journey. They are in the trenches every day, sometimes

working as late as 11 pm and on Saturdays, just trying to find the one key to unlocking a new

drug. Their research requires funding and most of that funding comes from the federal

government in the form of the National Institutes of Health (NIH). In 2013, the NIH appropriated

109 million dollars into the U.S. for research on lupus. But not all of Stefania's budget comes

from the NIH. About a quarter of her budget comes from private donors like the Lupus

Foundation of America (LFA). When I mentioned the CEO of the LFA, Annette Myarick, to

Stefania she had nothing but admiration.

"Of course I remember Annette. The grant from her foundation was the first grant I

received after arriving at CHOP (Children's Hospital of Philadelphia at the University of

Pennsylvania), and I always remember her foundation with gratitude. She came to bring me the check, in huge form, like 4x2ft. She took the picture of the two of us with the big check," Stefania said in an email.

When I went to meet Annette for the first time at the headquarters just outside of Philadelphia, she explained that helping up and coming researchers is where the foundation focuses. LFA feels it can do the most by supporting new researchers so they stay in the field of lupus research. It obviously worked out well in Stefania's case, since she continued lupus research in the decade following.

Meeting Annette at the LFA headquarters I also ran into a volunteer for the foundation, Cheri Perron. Cheri Perron was dressed all in purple the day I met her. It complemented her chocolate smooth skin. She carried a purple purse, wore a purple coat and atop her head was a purple knit hat. She wore a purple sweater and looked at the time on her purple watch.

"Purple was always my favorite color, but now I wear it for different reasons," she said. The Lupus Foundation of America has designated purple for lupus awareness and as a sufferer of lupus Cheri is like the poster child for advocacy.

Cheri talks with an air of assertiveness. When she speaks you listen. She has that concerned mother feel. You believe her when she described covering up with a big round hat and sunscreen, braving the sun, lupus's worst enemy, to watch her son's track meets. You believe her when she described fighting through the fatigue to see her daughter's ballet recitals. When I met her I was never so mindful of the words leaving my mouth. She annunciated each word she said and she spoke with impeccable grammar. But her formality did not overshadow her kindness. As an active volunteer for Lupus Foundation of America she embodies what it means to serve a cause. And she lives her cause every day with the never abating threat of kidney failure lurking around the corner. Forty percent of those with lupus will develop nephritis, or kidney inflammation.

When I began meeting patients and others involved with lupus I turned to the first person I'd think to talk to about it with- my uncle. As a primary care physician, he sees a wide range of ailments including lupus. The best way he described lupus to me was that it was a vascular and arthritic disease. It is a vascular disease because the immune system attacks the blood vessels. There are many blood vessels that go to different organs of the body so this can cause organ problems like kidney failure. It is arthritis because the immune system attacks the collagen of the joints and creates pain throughout the body.

### Inside the World of Kidney Nephritis

Let's take a moment and think about the world as a typical patient with lupus. One day you are going about your normal activities, food shopping, going to the gym, watching a favorite sitcom or taking care of your kids. For a few days you have experienced some pain in your joints and were more tired than usual but nothing you couldn't excuse. Pain? Maybe overdid it at the gym. Tired? Maybe not enough sleep. Then one day your feet and ankles swell up to the size of small melons and you are sent to the hospital. They run blood test after test and give you the one word diagnosis: lupus. Specifically, your kidneys are inflamed which is called lupus nephritis.

You might find yourself at the Lupus Foundation of America. They have chapters all across the United States. The Philadelphia Tri-State Chapter has headquarters right outside Philadelphia in Jenkintown, Pa. The first thing you notice when you step inside is the color purple. Just as pink is the badge of honor for those fighting breast cancer, purple is designated for lupus. A volunteer might greet you. She might even be Cheri Perron. If so, she would be dressed in her usual colors, all in purple, to promote self-advocacy. Annette Myarick, CEO of the chapter offers a handshake and the warmest smile you've ever seen. They say you are not alone. So many people suffer with lupus and so many others have no idea what it is. You're relieved you're not the only one who doesn't even know much about lupus. After they sit and talk with you about your diagnosis they give you a purple sack filled with pamphlets, magazines and business cards all centering around your disease.

Your disease. You don't like the implications of that two word phrase. At home the purple bag with the side that reads "Help Us Solve the Cruel Mystery. Lupus Foundation of America Philadelphia Tri-state Chapter," faces up on the bed. You stare at the cloth bag, unsure if you should dig into its contents. "Your disease." Did it define you now? What if you didn't want this disease? What did it mean about how you would live life from this moment onward? Would it ever go away?

You decide to go through the contents. You turn the purple bag upside down where you sit on the bed. First is a letter from Annette, the CEO with a warm smile. Key words pop out like "uncertainty" and "heartache" and "cruel mystery." You shuffle through to the "Lupus Now" magazine with a picture of Nick Cannon on the front. Intrigued, you turn to his story. He suffered from kidney nephritis as well, and he is a successful radio host, DJ, TV host, father, husband and more. As the host of America's Got Talent, he is the epitome of a healthy man, with a sleek suit, and a Hollywood smile. You start to skim but are pulled in by his story, so similar to your own. You remember somewhere in the past Nick Cannon stated he had a "lupus- like" disease, but here in this article he was coming right out and calling it lupus. The article explains how others advised him not to share his disease with the public because it might affect his work.

You can relate. There is no way you are telling the boss or anyone else at work you have a chronic illness. At least that's what the next pamphlet calls it, a chronic illness.

You remember Cheri, the volunteer from the LFA who shared her story with you. She said that she had lupus for quite a few years and then it was in 2001 the kidney problems really began. She woke up one Sunday morning ready for church. She was an active member. The mother of two and a woman with a successful career, she was always involved. Instead, this morning she felt dizzy and nauseous. She developed headaches, fatigue and extreme swelling in her feet. Her husband and kids watched as she was admitted to the hospital. They knew she had lupus, but for five years it had pretty much left her alone. She had fought, but now it seemed the lupus was winning. As Cheri's feet swelled, the signs of what was ailing her became clear. Her immune system was attacking the blood vessels of the kidney. The blood vessels were then leaking proteins out of the blood. Protein is very important for regulating the pressure of blood. Massive loss of protein causes the osmotic pressure in the capillaries to decrease, which causes fluid to flow out of the capillary and into the tissues causing edema, or swelling. Her kidneys were losing function and quickly. She had lost 90 % of her kidney function. In just a couple of days she went from a healthy active woman to someone who now faced being put on a waiting list for a kidney transplant.

She didn't need one. After high doses of chemotherapy drugs her immune system was suppressed enough that it no longer attacked her kidneys. To a point. Even today, thirteen years later, she says they still function at 65 to 70 percent.

You look again inside the purple bag. There are six "fact sheets" all about your disease:

- "What I need to know."
- "What I need to know about how lupus is diagnosed."

- "What I need to know about how lupus is treated"

- "How lupus may affect my body."

- "How lupus may affect my life."

- "Lupus and clinical depression."

Out of all of these you are most interested in what lupus is and the treatment. You want

to be cured. But the word *chronic* keeps appearing. It becomes clear there is no cure. One

patient said you have to manage the disease, see the doctor periodically and keep taking the

medication. For someone who has trouble taking Tylenol for a headache, taking medication for

the rest of your life is a huge blow. Another patient wrote of extreme fatigue; just getting a load

of laundry from the washer to the dryer made her out of breath. Other symptoms were scaly

rashes that could lead to hair loss. But the overall complaint was pain -- unrelenting pain caused

by the inflammation of the joints from the overactive immune system. You read about one

patient who wrote that her sister's advice was "it could be worse." You know this sentiment all

too well. On those days when you were so fatigued you couldn't get out of bed, your spouse

didn't understand and your kids couldn't help but need you to feel better. It wasn't until the

hospital stay that others noticed. And now that your kidney was in danger of failing it has kept

their attention.

But what to do about a failing kidney? The pamphlet's main answer is

immunosuppressive drugs and steroids. Corticosteroids like prednisone help with inflammation

of the kidney and joints but your eye quickly picks up on side effects- changes in appearance

such as acne or a round face and weight gain due to increased appetite and water retention. They

can also cause irritability, agitation, excitability or depression. It might sound vain, but you

don't want these effects. You don't want acne or to gain weight. As you read further about the immunosuppressive drugs such as Cytoxan you realize these are chemotherapy drugs and the side effects largely include hair loss and increased risk of infection. With the immune system suppressed, the antibodies of the immune system don't attack the kidney, but they also don't attack foreign viruses or bacteria so infection risk is high. You read on to find out infection is one of the leading causes of death in people with lupus. A bit of good news though. In another leaflet, Dr. Michael P. Madaio, M.D., who used to be the chief of nephrology and professor of medicine at Temple University, notes that CellCept, or mycophenolate mofetil, has fewer side effects and is as effective as steroids with immunosuppressive drugs.

Imagine how you feel at this point. Scared. Alone. Unsure. You've just stepped into the shoes of someone newly diagnosed with lupus, in particular lupus nephritis. I tried to imagine I was in the patient's shoes when Cheri handed me the purple bag full of information. Even though I was there to interview her about her experience with lupus nephritis and I myself did not have lupus, I could pretend that this was all happening to me, and it was overwhelming. Systemic lupus erythematosus is just as it says, it is systemic, or everywhere. The patient's autoantibodies attack joints and cause pain, they attack the central nervous system and cause numbness; they attack the blood vessels and cause organ failure or heart attacks.

****

Kidney failure is not the only result from lupus, but it is prevalent. The kidney is the size of a large orange and in such high demand that 106,000 Americans wait for one each year. It looks like the bean that bears its name. Place your hands on your hips and your thumbs that extend around to the back are touching the pair of them. The kidney, that small but fierce organ, is an underappreciated hero. Everyone always pays homage to the heart, but the kidneys are the powerhouse, the workhorse of the body and without them you're as good as dead. Every single minute of the day the kidneys receive one liter of blood. That means, if you were a kidney, the equivalent of drinking one glass every 15 seconds. The kidney filters 1500 liters of blood a day. Once it is inflamed by an autoimmune disease like lupus all bets are off and it begins to lose function.

Wenhai Shao, of Temple University, was purposely trying to inflame his kidneys. Not *his* kidneys per se, but the kidneys of the mice he was studying. He made a blood serum called nephrotoxic serum. When taken it induces kidney nephritis, or inflammation of the kidney that leads to kidney failure. To create the serum he sent pieces of the deceased mouse kidney to a company that injected it into a sheep. The sheep's immune system saw the kidney as foreign and created antibodies against the mouse kidney. When Wenhai injected the sheep serum full of antibodies against mouse kidney into a different healthy mouse, the antibodies attacked the mouse's kidney and caused kidney nephritis.

Real kidney nephritis, the kind not induced by a serum, works in a similar way.

"Lupus patients form immune complexes," Wenhai, a research scientist who worked under Dr. Philip Cohen at Temple University, explained to me one day in his office. "Immune complexes occur when the patient's antibodies bind to his own dead cells. They attach to the glomerulus of the kidney, or a network of capillaries that filter the blood, and cause kidney failure."

Later that day I sat on my bed with the "Textbook of Anatomy and Physiology" on my lap. Flipping to the back I recited the alphabet out loud to locate the letter K, a fourth grade habit I can't seem to kick. Kidneys, 446-458. Good sign. There were more than ten pages devoted to the topic. Before long I found myself drawing and labeling feverishly in a spiral bound notebook as I used to do in every single biology class I'd ever taken as an undergrad. The drawing staring back at me resembled the plumbing of the kitchen sink. I had drawn a nephron. We can all agree that one million is a big number. There are 2.5 million nephrons located in one kidney. A nephron is where the kidney's major function, the filtering of blood, takes place. The plumbing of the nephron started at the top called the glomerulus. It looked like a brain with a maze of capillaries that looked like worms. The heart pumps blood at such high pressure into the capillaries that water and nutrients are squeezed out of the "brain" glomerulus and into tubules. The tubule dipped down like a U, just as with the plumbing of a sink. The tubule goes down and comes back up and replenishes the blood with the water and nutrients that were taken away. Wastes like ammonia are secreted to a collecting duct, think of it as the bottom of a septic tank, and then to the ureters and out of the body as urine. One hundred and eighty quarts of blood a day are filtered to yield one and a half quarts of urine.

Wenhai had the nephrotoxic serum in his hand. He could induce mice to have kidney nephritis, or inflammation that is seen in patients with lupus. But what to do with it? It was like a jigsaw puzzle of pieces that if moved to the correct position would open up a bigger picture. The cell receptor called the Mer receptor was the key to that picture.

I met Wenhai Shao in the Health and Sciences building at Temple University on a cold day in late December. Stefania's group worked on the 11th floor and Wenhai worked for Dr. Philip Cohen on the fourth. Both were studying lupus. Wenhai was from a town outside Shanghai. He was a small framed man with small framed glasses, wispy black hair and a thick Asian accent. Love of his research, though, needed no translation.

"One time I bred one-hundred mice to get just one double knock-out that I needed for an experiment."

Wenhai hadn't bred a double knock out, or the deletion of two genes from the mouse

DNA code. It was a routine day in the lab in 2010 and he had bred Mer knock-out mice, which meant the mice didn't have any Mer receptors. When he compared normal mice with mice without Mer, he found that normal mice had high levels of Mer in the glomerulus of the kidney. This was the first time a study showed significant Mer receptors in the glomerulus. A major form of nephritis in lupus patients is *glomerulonephritis,* in which the glomerulus is damaged. Since Wenhai found Mer in the glomerulus, he thought it must be involved in kidney damage seen in lupus patients.

When Wenhai gave the nephrotoxic serum to normal mice he saw more Mer on the kidney. The mouse was producing more Mer in response to the deadly serum! These mice lived longer than mice that didn't have Mer. Somehow Mer stopped the damage from the antibodies of the nephrotoxic serum. Further, Wenhai found that Mer stopped the production of some of the cytokines like MCP-1, which are proteins that cause inflammation. The bigger picture was coming into focus. Perhaps if researchers could find a way to activate Mer in patients with lupus then there would be less inflammation and damage from antibodies of their immune system. It's one small step, but that is what so much of research is. It's trying to put the pieces of the puzzle together to find a therapy or medicine that will make the difference.

# 9. It Takes Two

Dear Diary 6/24/06

"I believe my illness is a blessing of sorts. In a former life I must have been a good person. This disease has forced me to refocus my life in a direction to help others within my limitations. This obstacle has forced me to creatively and whole-heartedly explore other areas for philanthropy. I could live without the ever-present pain, though, without the pain there would be no relief." – Erin Castaldi

To Elizabeth and Robert Lowell, March 17, 1953

"I am making out fine in spite of any conflicting stories. I have a disease called lupus and I take medicine called ACTH and I manage well enough to live with both. Lupus is one of those things in the rheumatic department; it comes and goes, when it comes I retire and when it goes, I venture forth. My father had it some twelve or fifteen years ago but at that time there was nothing for it but the undertaker; now it can be controlled with the ACTH. I have enough energy to write with and as that is all I have any business doing anyhow, I can with one eye squinted take it all as a blessing. What you have to measure out, you come to observe closer, or so I tell myself." – Flannery O'Connor

\*\*\*\*

Ten years ago Uma never expected to be emotionally attached to her work and her colleague, Stefania halfway across the world from where she grew up.

"It's been a long journey. Ten years we've worked together. That's a long time," Uma said.

To say that Stefania and Uma are on the same page is an understatement. They can finish each other's sentences and ideas. They are both have degrees in immunology and both wear their dark hair in ponytails. For a little more than a decade they have worked together focused on dendritic cells in autoimmunity. Uma grew up in Chennai, India; Stefania outside Rome, Italy. Both are passionate about the same things- research on one hand and teaching on the other. Although Uma is not a professor at Temple like Stefania, her love of teaching is apparent in the lab. Most days she's mentoring the other PhD candidates: Marita, Jun, Paul and Rob.

"She has a base knowledge that we can tap into easily when she's there. She's always willing to help," Paul said.

Although petite and soft spoken, when she speaks it is with conviction and confidence. She listens patiently to their concerns and step by step calmly explains how to proceed. That much has not changed since I worked with her at University of Pennsylvania. No matter how many times I asked the same question, and I repeatedly asked many of the same questions, she would respectfully answer it like it was the first time being asked.

When I asked her what brought her to the United States I was expecting the classic answer about funding.

"Yes, you're right there is more funding for research here in the United States, but it wasn't so much the funding as much as I wanted more knowledge to take back with me to India so I could teach more students," Uma explained. "Right now, it is a good situation for research in India because most of the pharma is being outsourced there. Many of my colleagues have gone back. But I'm not sure if I'd go back. I have a green card now."

Uma's original plans were not to work for big pharma in India. After her masters degree in zoology from Madras University in India, she took a placement test. Her score determined if she could pursue both research and a lectureship. Uma scored high. She was eligible to teach.

No matter if for money or not, that was what she wanted more than anything else.

"I volunteered to teach many times at the college."

"My daughter says she's proud of me. I used to teach a lot in India. I ran a night school out of my house. Kids of all ages in neighborhood came. The school started at the 10th grade level. I used to teach summer courses for placement/entrance exams and I coached for the life sciences exam. Students needed a certain score to get to college. I did it for free for many kids. I used to take fees if they really wanted it -- only if I knew they could afford it"

It is that same warm-hearted spirit that gives Uma her charm. By spending just one day in the lab with her one would immediately notice that warmth extends to her both her families- her lab family and her family outside the lab as well. She is in awe of her young seven- year old only child, Soumya. Most nights after coming home from work she sits and has tea with Soumya while doing homework together. Uma mentioned Soumya periodically as she worked.

"Did you know about these rainbow loom jewelry?" Uma said with a slight Indian accent.

I shook my head no.

"It's the latest trend with children. It's these different color rubber bands that she braids together. It's from a rainbow loom kit. My house is like a rainbow loom factory! I think the other week I spent $40 dollars just in rubber bands!" Uma gets a kick out of it all as she laughs with her whole body. Her laughs are infectious, ranging from a low giggle at times to a deep chuckle.

She sets the tone of the entire lab. Her laugh just makes you feel good. And it's more than just the laugh. Not only is she in charge of managing the lab supply, she is a reservoir of knowledge for the PhD candidates and even for Stefania. She has made lupus her life's work and it shows.

Stefania is right there behind her. She is the support for all of her lab members and has made lupus her life's work as well. At 11:00 on Monday morning she sat down with Paul for their weekly meeting. Next to her were filing cabinets with a magnet that held up the note: "Jun Xu Aug 14, Paul May 15, Marita Aug 15.

"I keep a note on when my students are graduating," Stefania explained. She was as invested in their future as they were.

"So what do you want to talk about," she asked.

Paul seemed quite relaxed, leaning back in his chair as he spoke. It was obvious to me that Stefania provided a working environment that fostered trust and a degree of calmness. She wasn't out to break her students down. Quite the contrary, she was out to help them reach their goals.

As they talked, Stefania steered the conversation like an expert. She asked questions to lead Paul to his own answers. I felt I was watching an expert teacher work. The conversation invariably shifted to the Curli experiments. Curli was the bacteria he had shown might induce autoimmunity like lupus.

"The mice still aren't showing proteinuria, or protein in the urine," Paul shook his head and let out an "I just don't know" laugh.

Stefania was unintimidated. As was her style she had an answer.

"I have doubt. It could be our animal facility delays proteinuria. Let's run a control the same way I did the experiments when I was at Children's Hospital at University of Penn. If we don't get proteinuria then we know we have a problem," she said.

On Tuesday morning it was Jun's turn to meet with Stefania. Stefania pulled up the graph results of her experiments on the computer screen. They sat and starred at the screen and just thought.

Stefania said, "The graphs are beautiful," and then they sat and stared some more. Then as she always does Stefania came up with a new direction for the research.

"It would be interesting to see if the difference between female and male is in terms of suppressor cells. There is some literature saying there is a difference in suppressor cells between males and females," Stefania said.

Stefania is like a walking library of literature on dendritic cells and the immune system. If there was a paper written having the slightest bit to do with her experiments she probably read it and could recite the findings. That is what makes her and her team work so well together. Her students are on the floor doing the experiments day in and day out, and she can view their results and put together a plan on what to target and where to focus. That is exactly what funding institutions like the LFA are hoping for. That is why they fund young researchers like they did with Stefania some ten years ago. They bet on the idea that they will push the field of lupus research forward, and many like Stefania have.

# 10. Annette and Cheri – Dedicated to the LFA

Dear Diary 5-17-10

"The Walk for Lupus Now 2010 turned out to be a great day. When the last person arrived in the morning we tallied the money at $325. Everyone chipped in. We had 14 friends and family on team Butterfly Warriors. I have such a supportive and loving family. Everyone had to plan and organize [sic] their life around this event. I feel blessed that so many people would change and set aside their morning for me. It was a blast."—Erin Castaldi

Discoveries, like Wenhai's of the potential benefits of the Mer receptor, or Uma's of the role of TLR 7 and TLR 9 in lupus do not just happen. The researchers at Temple, like researchers in universities across the nation, need to be funded and supported.

Maybe you're one of the lucky ones, one of the ones who do not need to rely on the advances of medicine. Then again, maybe you're one of the seventy percent of Americans, according to CBS News, that take prescription drugs. If you're one of the 1.5 million Americans with lupus you need medication more than ever. But it's not just lupus. It's everything. From depression to heart disease to asthma to diabetes, we rely on our biomedical industry that touts its success on the National Institutes of Health (NIH) website. There, in big bold letters, the site says that the average life span increases by one year every six years due to their research.

The NIH is the largest source of funding for biomedical research in the United States, funding about 90% of all research. The funds go to over 300,000 research personnel at more than 2,500 universities and research institutions throughout the United States, according to the NIH website. An upwards of seventy percent of Stefania's budget comes from the NIH which is directly supported by government funding. So it's not like if all of a sudden the NIH lacked funds to support Stefania that she would be unaffected. Quite the contrary, she would be affected very much. Although 109 million dollars for lupus research seems like a lot, it must be shared over multiple universities and multiple labs throughout the country. And with the price of one molecular biology reagent for Stefania's research costing 1500 dollars, it is easy to see how money can be tight.

Money is the driving force behind private institutions such as the LFA, as well. I went back to LFA headquarters later in the month to follow up with Cheri and Annette and see how things were going.

On the wall at their Philadelphia headquarters, was a framed "Lupus Now" Magazine cover. It showed a big number 10 for ten year anniversary edition. I remembered it from the materials Cheri handed me in the purple bag when I first met her and Annette at the Lupus Foundation of America Tristate headquarters near Philadelphia. Today, I was staying in the waiting area. Cheri hadn't arrived yet. I was there to continue our interview from our first meeting. Instead, I met Annette, who was in good spirits as usual. Although she was half hidden behind mounds of paper on her desk and although when I asked her what was on the agenda for today she had to take a breath in before letting the list roll, she still smiled between every other sentence.

"Well, what is there NOT to do, that is the question," Annette said with a chuckle. "Let's see, so we do everything here from strategic thinking to data entry. Right now I'm trying to lock down locations for training of our support leaders. Also we are working on launching the New Jersey and Delaware walk campaigns."

"I am about to be in a conference call with Leila, a board member who will be development committee chairperson. Cheri is supposed to be on the call too, but she is running late," Annette said. She explained that Cheri was still at her doctor's appointment.

Not too long ago I had to go to the doctor's for a small hiccup to my system. It was in no way as serious as lupus, but I was nervous none the less. Having interviewed patients with lupus these past few months, I was used to being on the other side of things. I had even felt what it was like being a doctor in a lupus ward at the hospital. Now I was escorted back to a small room with Pepto-Bismol colored walls where I waited. A young resident, dressed much the way I had been at Temple Hospital with the lab coat and all, asked me questions that not too long ago I had observed being asked of lupus patients.

"Shortness of breath?"

"No."

"Dizziness?"

"No."

"Hair loss?"

"No."

I wasn't being treated for lupus, but I had the weird sensation of seeing everything from outside myself. Not too long ago I had donned the lab coat and followed Dr. Caricchio around as he gave out either good or bad news. I wanted to tell the young doctor, "I was you. I played the part of a resident just like you a few weeks ago." Now I was the nervous one awaiting news from a different doctor.

Either way I felt for Cheri. Going to the doctor's when you have lupus must be far from a stress-free event.

Annette continued speaking, bringing me back from my thoughts.

"We have a board meeting next Wednesday. I need to review audited financial statements of 2013. We need to budget more conservatively this year than last year. It's the first time in my history that we have a 50,000 deficit," Annette said.

As was her style, she found the silver lining in what she said. Although their budget shrank the year the economy tanked, they had been trying to make up ground ever since 2008 and today the NIH put out a press release stating the LFA along with other nonprofits, ten biopharmaceutical companies and the NIH will all collaborate to find new drugs targeted at Alzheimer's disease, type 2 diabetes, rheumatoid arthritis and lupus. The government funded the project $230 million dollars. The press release said currently developing a drug from discovery through to FDA approval takes over a decade and failure rate is more than 95%. Each success costs more than $1 billion dollars. If the big pharma and NIH research institutes collaborate it might speed up the process.

Cheri was taking two drugs: CellCept and Plaquenil, both not specific for lupus. The first works on suppressing the immune system and the second to help stop a lupus flare and help with skin issues. Only one drug in fifty years, Benlysta, had been brought to market specifically for lupus.

We started the conference call without Cheri. As Annette searched for certain missing papers in the stacks on her desk, her assistant took notes. Both listened to Leila and it was clear that their task would be to drum up sponsors for the upcoming walks and events. Midway through the meeting Cheri made it in.

"How are you Cheri?" asked Leila through the speaker phone.

"Oh it's another day. It's another day," Cheri sighed.

Cheri sat down and began to take notes – with her purple pen. I remembered how everything of hers was purple the last time I saw her but I was amazed at how many more of her things were actually that color. There was the pen and then I saw earrings I didn't notice the first time. Plus she was writing on a purple notepad. It was impressive to be so open and dedicated to one's cause.

At the conclusion of the conference call, the three women in the office began hashing out everyone's job in creating sponsors. Everyone wanted to be clear on exactly what had to be done. After only spending 45 minutes with the group I wished I could help in some way. Their spirit was infectious.

In the hallway I asked Cheri what she meant earlier by, "It's another day."

"Oh I guess I should be grateful. I am grateful, but it's never easy when I see my rheumatologist," she said.

"Oh?" I asked.

"Yes, I am trying to get off medication and my doctor wants to add medication or keep me on what I'm taking."

"That must be frustrating," I said.

"Yes it is," Cheri said. "Now, how can I help you today?"

"I just wanted to know what you normally do when you come to the LFA office."

"Well I start by checking the Phone Call Literature Request. There are Client Intake forms that are filled out for people who have reached out to us. I follow up with them and call them and answer any questions and I send them a packet like the one I gave you."

"I guess today you'll also be working on setting up new sponsors?" I asked.

"Yes, I'll be on the computer most of the day," Cheri said.

Our conversation veered from her volunteer responsibilities to her love of Edgar Allen Poe to her addiction to James Patterson crime novels. There was no doubt she was a well-read woman. I told her I was going to the lupus walk coming up this year and that made her smile. Then all of a sudden her smile grew.

"I have *purple bubbles!* I bought them especially for the lupus walk!" she said.

Purple bubbles. Now I definitely had to walk.

The next few hours Cheri and the other few women at LFA would be on the computer scouring the internet for would-be sponsors for the upcoming lupus walks they were organizing. It was clear that they never gave up. No matter what the economic climate they pushed on, just as Cheri pushed on with the hopes of living without the side effects of her medication. They were relentless, relentless in their fight for their cause, and relentless in their personal fights against the disease.

# 11. Funding Problems

Dear Diary, 1/14/12

"I have gained so much weight from the steroids these past few months. Probably about 20 lbs! Surprising. I just noticed 1 day that I couldn't fit in my skinny jeans and my fat jeans fit perfectly. This not O.K. I don't like the feel of my body w/ this extra weight SO. .. I have cut out all sugar in my diet ... My clothes will fit again!" – Erin Castaldi

To Janet McKane, June 19, 1963

"The self-portrait was made ten years ago, after a very acute siege of lupus. I was taking [the steroid] cortisone which gives you what they call a moon-face and my hair had fallen out due to a large extent from the high fever, so I looked pretty much like the portrait. When I painted it I didn't look at myself in the mirror ... I knew what [I] looked like." – Flannery O'Connor


\*\*\*\*


I continued to follow everyone I interviewed, from the researchers, to the patient, to charitable organizations like the LFA. I tried to follow up with Paul on his research showing that Curli can cause lupus in mice. His was the first presentation I saw when I arrived at Temple and I was curious how the research was going. Up until this point he hadn't seen any proteins in the urine, a symptom of the disease. I followed up on this point with him as the weeks progressed. One week later, then two weeks later I emailed him asking if proteins showed in the urine. At first he said no, that he had detected no proteins. I later caught up with him in the lab. He explained how they get the urine from each mouse by massaging the bladder. There are special cages to collect the urine but the researchers here didn't use them. I belabored my same question about proteins in the urine once more. Paul sighed heavily.

"No they're not showing protein," he said.

In the break room Uma, the senior researcher who had worked with Stefania for 10 years, suggested that such a result might mean the mice are showing a different autoimmune disease and not lupus. The work was not over for Paul. He would have to be diligent and follow up his results with even more testing. PCR, ELISA, Flow cytommetry, Western blot. These unfamiliar words to us make up Paul's life. He performs these tests Monday through Friday, and most Saturdays.

"I come in to the lab on Saturdays because it's easier to run a full test from start to end with no distraction," Paul said to me one day while taking a break from the lab.

Paul embodied everything you would expect of a scientist.

"As a kid I loved nature. I loved backpacking, hiking, and climbing. I used to like learning about trees. I guess that's where I learned to enjoy being a 'naturalist,'" Paul said.

As it should be with any budding science PhD candidate, Paul is a fan of *Dr. Who* and *The Hitchhiker's Guide to the Galaxy*, the book, not the movie of course. I could tell after just a few minutes talking to him that he was right where he belonged.

"I was almost a philosophy major, then English or politics. Then I had taken an introductory biology course and learned about genes -- it blew my mind how it works," Paul said.

It's that fascination that drives him to faithfully continue his experiments day after day and to persist when the results are not what he expects. And most times the results are unexpected.

"That's the beauty of science. You have to figure out why the results are the way they are," Paul explained.

When I shadowed Uma in the lab the next week, she and the PhD student Marita unknowingly agreed with Paul's sentiment. I was back in the lab observing everyone at work.

"All right Uma Guma, how's it going?"

"She calls me Uma Guma," Uma chuckled.

"Isn't that like a Pink Floyd album or something?" Marita said.

Uma and Marita work on opposite sides of the lab bench in Stefania's lab.

"So what is the most challenging thing about being a PhD student?" I asked.

"Patience. It teaches you patience." Marita said

Uma smiled and nodded her head up and down a few times.

"That is so true," she said.

"And a lot of perseverance. Every time you think you should give up you have to be resilient," Marita added.

Perseverance. Uma has worked her results ten times over in order to submit her findings for her latest experiment with TLRs. It came down to the wire and she enlisted the help of other members of the lab like Jun to finalize graphs and figures. She asked if she could have the best graphs for the IL-4 data. Jun asked her to clarify. With her reading glasses perched on the top of her jet black ponytail, Uma spoke calmly but firmly. She explained,

"I just need the graph. Export it as a Tif file, take it to the power point and see how it looks." There is a way that Uma has when giving direction that signifies without a doubt she's the senior scientist in the lab. One moment she can be assertive, giving direction, and the next like a school girl giggling at herself or with others.

Perseverance. As Uma worked she explained how perseverance is not only needed in the lab but in the office as well. As the only PhD in the lab she worked closely with Stefania. She explained how every two or three years there is a crisis with funding.

"I've worked for her for 10 years. It has always worked out favorable; either she or I got the grant."

Stefania and Uma's salaries were totally dependent on the grants they received. Medical advance needs money and it needs money from the government. Private institutions themselves cannot pick up the slack from lack of government funding. The private institution Lupus Foundation of America has a yearly budget of $500,000 dollars. Only a fraction of the $500,000 dollars ends up with researchers like Stefania. The organization's entire budget equals the amount of money Stefania gets from one grant from the government and she gets multiple grants.

Mr. Stephen Ezell, an economist and senior analyst with the Information Technology and Innovation Foundation (ITIF) insists that government investment in research is also needed because private investment only blossoms with increases in government spending. He writes in his blog:

*Public and private investments in R&D are complementary. (In fact, research finds that each additional dollar of public contract research added to the stock of government R&D has the effect of inducing an additional 27 cents of private R&D investment.)*

In other words, private investment needs government spending.

There had been moments in Stefania and Uma's ten year history where they had experienced lack of grants from the NIH, but for some reason something always came through. This may have been true in the past, but it was becoming increasingly more and more difficult to just survive.

From 1998 to 2003 the NIH funding from the U.S. government doubled and then it plateaued without another real increase in the years to come. Because of inflation, the spending power of the dollar decreased, so the budget has been constantly eroding since 2003. Then came sequestration in 2013. Because Congress could not agree on a budget to reduce the national deficit, automatic cuts went into effect. The sequestration required the NIH to cut 5% or 1.55 billion dollars from its budget for the fiscal year 2013.

The sequester hurts researchers like Stefania. Multi-year grants that promised a certain set of money over the course of a few years were cut back. Instead of getting 100 percent of the grant they might only get 80 percent. With such large decreases, staff is usually cut. When I asked Stefania about the climate of being a researcher in 2014 she was less than enthusiastic.

"Many of my colleagues had to shut down their labs. There's just no money," she said.

Dr. Cohen, her colleague who supervises Wenhai Shao's research, said, "I don't know why scientists stay in the field. I don't know why people put up with this kind of life. It's really very stressful."

For many researchers not yet tenured, their salary and the salaries of those in their lab are totally dependent on getting funded from outside institutions. Principal investigators, or research scientists who run labs, like Stefania, go from grant to grant year after year, applying for new grants to fund themselves and their research. But year after year she pushes through. As labs are closing around her, Stefania hasn't given up her pursuits of understanding lupus eventually finding a cure.

# 12. An Unwelcome Goodbye

Dear Diary, 9/21/08

"I feel like I am in mourning, but for what? My health, a career never explored, unexpected financial burdens that I am unable to help fix. I have a chronic fear of inevitable pain. It's there lying in the wait for me like a snake under a log. Quiet, steady, can wait as long as I can. Always pokes its head out to show me his power and my place in his world."

To "A" December 24, 1960

What they found out at the hospital is that my bone disintegration is being caused by the steroid drugs which I have been taking for ten years to keep the lupus under control. So they are going to try to withdraw the steroids and see if I can get along without them. If I can't, as Dr. Merril says, it is better to be alive with joint trouble than dead without it. Amen..." – Flannery O'Connor

\*\*\*\*

I took the elevator to the 11th floor as I usually did and walked down the hall to Stefania's office. As normal, she was fixated on the computer screen in front of her. I knocked and said good morning. Something was off. Stefania seemed preoccupied. As we talked the discussion invariably steered to the topic of funding.

"I don't like how it's all about money now. It used to be about interesting things like science," she said.

"Well it seems like you're doing ok. You have a lot of people working for you in the lab."

Stefania looked perplexed and upset at the same time.

"You don't know?"

Know what? I thought.

"I had to let Uma go."

The words hit like mallets striking my chest. I took a deep breath. How could this happen? Stefania said there's just no money, but still, didn't Uma just say there was a crisis every few years and it always turned out favorably? Uma was being let go and she never told me.

I made my way to the break area and was about to put my lunch in the refrigerator when Uma came around the corner. She baked muffins as she always did, microwaved one and offered it to me. I ate it not sure what to say.

"Do you taste the secret ingredient? It's love," Uma said, drawing out the word.

She was still jocular even in spite of her current circumstances.

"I have news to tell you. It changes everything. We must talk," she said.

"I think I already know Uma. Stefania told me … when is your last day?" I asked

"Friday."

Friday. Only four days away. Ten years and in only four days it was over. Never mind how crushed I felt for her. I wondered how she was feeling. Could I have one last interview with her here in the lab?

"Certainly, let me take care of some stuff and we'll talk," Uma said.

Back in the lab Jun sits at the computer next to Uma. Both talk quietly. Uma says she is proud she stayed with almost no funding.

"It's a long investment of time you know?" Uma said.

Jun just nods. Uma is quiet.

All of a sudden Uma is excited.

"Marie got back to me!" she said to the others in the lab.

Marita, Jun and Rob huddled around Uma's computer screen

"We've reviewed your proposal and your work is outstanding. Your grant has been reviewed and received a score of 21. Please note our council does not make funding decisions per se. It's possible that the pay line won't be established until after the council meets. It's also possible that the initial pay line will be set low and perhaps even go up towards the end of the fiscal year. The council meets in February," Uma read from the computer screen.

"See this is why I like Marie as the council director. She called my work outstanding!" Uma said.

"That's great Uma Guma!!" Marita said.

"Yeah that's awesome," Rob added.

What does this mean?

Uma's proposal for a grant from the government agency NIH received a score of 21 with 10 being the best score at 10 and around 100 being the worst. With her score there is a chance she could be approved for the grant in February, which means if she applied to work in other labs she would be bringing 30-40 % of her salary, already paid for, and contributing at least 20 % of the grant money to the lab itself.

Some of her colleagues had advised Uma to leave the profession, but with her score of 21 Uma is heartened. She did toy with the idea of medical writing instead of research, but research is where she lives. To push on, even when it seems like everything is against her, is who she is.

# 13. Feeling the Effects of Dwindling Funds

Dear Diary 4/7/14

Today I had plans with my uncle and it couldn't happen. I couldn't get out of bed. I couldn't keep my eyes open, my muscles hurt. It's like a tired you feel in your bones. Foggy brain and the whole thing. Sometimes I have extreme lethargy I just can't control. It's hard to explain to others.

To "A" November 16, 1957

Your visit was thoroughly enjoyed by us and is always good for me though I may look tired. The truth is I am tired every afternoon and there's nothing to be done about it. It's the nature of the disease. A lot of people decide I am bored or indifferent or uppity but at a certain hour of the day my motor cuts off automatically.


****


Although Uma doesn't plan on leaving the profession or on leaving the country, the research climate in the U.S. is causing many others to reconsider. I ran across a recent Business Insider article titled, "Why a Nobel Laureate is Telling his Students to go to other Countries." Dr. James Rothman, who won the prize in medicine, believes budget cuts make it more difficult for the US to retain the world's top science talent. He actually now tells his students to go abroad.

"I actually advise my students not to stay in the United States," he said. "Frankly if I were 10 years younger, that's exactly what I would do."

Leaving the United States is not an option for Uma. She devoted more than a decade here in the U.S. obtaining her green card and setting up residence outside Philadelphia and has no desire to give up everything she's worked for.

When I think of the United States in the world of life science I think of a behemoth. Actually when I think of the United States in any science I think of someone crushing the worldwide competition. But most of what we rely on today was set up decades ago and we are not keeping pace. I think it's hard for certain Congressmen to see the value in funding because the effect is not immediate. What makes it even more difficult is the political climate in which we exist, where Republicans and Democrats can't agree. However, it is possible for Republicans and Democrats to work together. They did in the past and can do it again. There had been, up until presently, a 15-year bipartisan support of biomedical research. Republicans that made it happen, like John Porter from Illinois, insist our economic destiny depends on funding science and technology, according to the New York Times.

Lawmakers met in January of 2014 to restore some of the funds cut by sequestration. The Health and Human Services appropriations committee (HHS) was a subcommittee formed to deal with budget allocations for groups like the NIH. They passed a two year budget deal which restored funding to 29.93 billion for 2014. It's a step in the right direction but far from perfect. I spoke with Dr. Carrie Wolinetz who serves as current President of United for Medical Research, a leading coalition of universities, patient groups, and private sector companies advocating for sustainable funding for the NIH. She explained that although it is a step in the right direction, it is just a Band-Aid and not a cure.

"To be fair the HHS appropriations subcommittee didn't get a lot to work with, but I think the reason that this is insufficient is because it didn't restore cuts of sequestration totally,"

Carrie said. "NIH got a billion dollars less than what was cut in sequestration. Plus, as a result of inflation we see a decline in the purchasing power, a 20 percent drop, for NIH and every dollar is going a little less far. If you take that into account with the sequester the budget deal didn't go far enough."

Dr. Daniel Raben, a professor of biochemistry at Johns Hopkins University School of Medicine, had to lay off a technician and a grad student due to lack of funding according to another Washington Post article. He was quoted as saying, "Instead of trying to think about the best science, [researchers] think about it as a business person. 'Where's the money? What's the question that I can ask that can get money?' And I find that to be very disheartening and even dangerous because we're not going to make progress that way."

Even if funding were restored to pre-sequester levels, the budget deal from January of 2014 does not reverse the pattern of America's dwindling role in the world of biomedical research. Dr. Francis Collins told the Atlantic that China is aiming to outspend the U.S. in the next five years – not as a percentage of GDP but in absolute dollars.

Stephen Ezell, an economist and senior analyst with the Information Technology and Innovation Foundation (ITIF), argues in his book *Innovation Economics* that true innovation can come from a balance between the public and private sectors and that both are needed to spur technological growth, but he does not minimize the role of government support in bringing important technologies to market.

"Research supported by the National Institutes of Health (NIH) practically created the U.S. biotechnology industry," Ezell writes. "And yes, even Google, the Web search darling, isn't a purebred creature of the free market; the search algorithm it uses was developed as part of the National Science Foundation (NSF) - funded Digital Library Initiative."

After reading Stephen Ezell's book I called him to clear up any confusion I had even on basic economics. To begin with I asked why are numbers presented as a share of the gross domestic product (GDP) and what does that mean? Ezell explained that you cannot represent how much the government is investing in the NIH as just dollars. It may look like it is the same amount this year as it was ten years ago but it is actually 22 % less because of inflation. That is why he talks about share of the GDP. We invest a quarter less of share of GDP than a decade ago.

"China will spend four times as much as share of GDP on biomedical research in next five years as us," Stephen Ezell said over the phone.

Ezell explained how lack of government funding in the biotech sector can have a ripple effect.

"There are two effects,"Ezell said. "First of all, the declining budget means fewer grants will get awarded. Second, the age of someone getting a grant has increased. It has increased substantially, actually. It has gone from 34 years old in 1970 to 42 in 2005. You tend to get riskier more innovative ideas from younger researchers, so less money means less innovative ideas. Plus, applicants for grants won't put forward their most innovative ideas because they are riskier and may not get funded."

A couple of months after Uma left Stefania's lab, Marita responded to my request and sent me pictures of Uma's last day. I wasn't around to see Uma off that day, but the pictures said everything I suspected. Uma smiled and held up a framed graph showing dendritic cell activation markers with the signature of everyone from the lab. And in the next photo she stood holding the graph next to the group of researchers all trying to find the same clue, the same cure. Uma would not give up. The photos showed that she meant to push on and that even if she had to stop researching lupus for a moment, she would be back at it the minute the opportunity arose. She would persevere.

# 14. Discoveries

Dear Diary, 12/1/10

"I want to continue tutoring, but need to keep this job. My body just hurts so bad after a shift I can't even do anything for 2-4 hours. Work has been excruciating. Either my right hip or low/mid back is cry worthy three quarters through a shift. I asked for 20 hrs max, but next week I'm on for 32 including flex. I am either recovering from or getting ready for work. No more walking through the mall before work and definitely no strolling after work." – Erin Castaldi

To Elizabeth Fenwick, February 12, 1954

"I am not able enough to walk straight but not crippled enough to walk with a cane so that I give the appearance of merely being a little drunk all the time. No spots or butterfly wings.[2]"
—Flannery O'Connor

\*\*\*\*

Published in 1973, Ralph Steinman wrote about what was a routine observation of mouse spleen cells. The spleen is where antibodies of the immune system are created. Back on that fateful day in the early 1970s, Steinman chopped the mouse spleen into fine chunks and then sieved them through a cell strainer. He disrupted the spleen further by sucking it up and then out several times with a pipette. Next he let the clumps of spleen settle and took the liquid on top of the clumps, the supernatant, and spun it in a centrifuge. The resulting cell pellet was re-suspended in blood serum from a cow. He put the spleen cell/serum mixture on glass cover slips and plastic petri dishes for one hour at 37 degrees. He expected to see all known kinds of cells adhere to the surface and he did. He observed granulocytes, a type of white blood cell,

---

[2] She is referencing the butterfly rash on the face common in patients with lupus.

lymphocytes, which are B and T lymphocytes that produce antibodies against foreign invaders, and mononuclear phagocytes, such as macrophages which directly digest cell debris and pathogens. What he didn't expect were cells with "pseudopods of various length, width, form and number," as he called them, or extensions out from the center of the cell like dendrites. The green stained cell extensions stared back at him through the light microscope. No one had identified such cells ever before. He wrote:

"These novel cells can assume a variety of branching forms, and constantly extend and retract many fine cell processes. The term 'dendritic' cell would thus be appropriate for this particular cell type."

The dendritic cell was born.

Steinman would later receive the 2011 Nobel prize in Physiology or Medicine for his discovery and work with dendritic cells. Ten years after his initial discover of dendritic cells, in 1983, he and colleagues Gutchinov, Witmer, and Nussenzweig, used an anti-dendritic cell antibody to kill dendritic cells and found that it reduced the immune response. In his famous review in 1998 with Jacques Banchereau they proposed that dendritic cells not only activate T lymphocytes which then induce B lymphocyte growth, but also directly activate B lymphocytes, which are cells producing antibodies against foreign invaders in the body. T and B lymphocytes are cells of the immune system that work together to produce antibodies that go on to kill pathogens. Steinman showed that the dendritic cell activates them. That paper was cited over a thousand times. Most scientists think they are rock stars when their papers are referenced a hundred times.

Dendritic cells take in what is called the antigen or a piece of the pathogen (for example a piece of a virus or bacterium) that they then present, or display, on the outside of their cell. That is why they are called antigen presenting cells (APCs). They present this antigen, or piece of the pathogen, to T lymphocyte in order to activate them. Once activated, the "helper" T lymphocytes, Th2 and Th1, go on to activate B lymphocytes, which produce antibodies to neutralize the pathogen by recognizing the same piece of the pathogen, the antigen that was presented by the dendritic cell.

Exactly forty years later, Jun, one of the researchers in Stefania's lab, owed her research to Dr. Steinman. If it wasn't for his discovery of the dendritic cell, she would not be studying dendritic cells' role in the disease lupus. But her studies hit an impasse. She sat in the Stefania's lab and poured over the multitude of recent papers on dendritic cells, but they contradicted her findings. She knew patients with active lupus have high levels of Type 1 Interferon, proteins that have been implicated in lupus. They are produced in large numbers by dendritic cells.

Jun sat quietly at her desk; the numbers on the green graph- lined paper of the notebook didn't make sense. She ran the numbers again. Jun's laboratory results were clear: high levels of Type I Interferon in dendritic cells meant high levels of TREX-1, another protein that has been implicated in lupus. All the papers suggested the opposite result. She had found a direct link between TREX-1and Type I Interferon. TREX-1 is thought to be involved with Erin's type of lupus where there are neurologic problems.

"Science is full of possibilities and impossibilities." June said. "You think it's almost not possible that it will work out and it does, or you think it's possible and it doesn't work. With TREX-1 the other studies made me think if I give Type I Interferon to the dendritic cells then TREX-1 would go down because it would be inhibited. That's not what happened. I thought, 'Did I do something wrong?' So I have to go back through all the literature again. It's all about not giving up. I didn't and there was a paper that supported my findings."

"TREX-1 has been implicated in neurological conditions with patients with particular forms of lupus," Jun said to me at the break table just outside the lab.

Google the TREX-1 gene and sure enough studies do connect lupus patients who have neurological symptoms to mutations in their TREX-1 gene. Jun's next challenge will be to show that dendritic cells from lupus mice have high levels of the TREX-1 gene and try and discover what it means about the disease.

Her research cannot come fast enough for patients like Erin Castaldi whose major symptoms are neurologic. Lupus attacks her central nervous system, causing the numbness down her left side and leading to her walking with a limp. Any bit closer to understanding the role of TREX-1 in lupus could mean one step closer to Erin walking without her cane. And just like Erin never gives up hope that she can lead a fulfilling life despite her illness, Jun has never given up the pursuit of a cure.

# 15. Beating the Odds

Dear Diary 2/8/06

"Well my hair has begun to get loose again. As w/ methotrexate it is no longer brushing out in 2-3 strands but small clumps of 5-10 + or more. If it comes out fully Paul said he would shave his head. He is tremendously thoughtful ... I feel like I have a time bomb inside of me and I just keep waiting for the "side effects" to begin. I have heard of so many terrible symptoms from the medicine and if they really are worse than those of methotrexate I'm not looking forward to them." – Erin Castaldi

To Maryat Lee July 1, 1964

"My dose of prednisone has been cut in half on Dr. Merrill's orders because the nitrogen content of the blood has increased by a third. So far as I can see the medicine and the disease run neck and neck to kill you, but anyway I don't hear any choruses now, no more 'Clementine' or 'Coming for to Carry Me Home.' I am likely some better" – Flannery O'Connor

\*\*\*\*

It was nine degrees outside, but the wind made it feel like one. Working outside when the temperature doesn't even reach double digits just seemed unnatural. Paul did it anyway. He had been on the clock for over 200 hours now, sleeping in intervals in the back of his truck. For months he had been used to working 80 hour/ 90 hour work weeks. Then back in January his boss asked him to take a special assignment to head up a job at the Sunoco Marcus Hook refinery, hauling butane from one side of the plant to the other. It was tedious work, but it paid four dollars an hour more with unlimited hours. When forced to decide, he focused on his wife Erin's smile. She was worth it. Everything she had been through and everything they had been through together was worth their planned adventure. And they needed money to see this adventure through. A year long cross -country road trip is not cheap and so Paul pushed through wanting to quit. There was no quitting. Erin needed a change of scenery, and he was there to offer it to her.

Erin has always relished adventure. She liked to do things outside the norm. She liked to push herself. Erin was obsessed with joining the Peace Corps, almost blind to the fact that most likely the Peace Corps would not accept a patient with an illness like her's. All she could focus on was that one dream. When it wasn't coming true, she didn't give up, but rather pursued a cross-country road trip. That is why Paul gave up working on his small business and went back to work full-time to raise the money to fund the trip. At the end of the first two weeks at his new position, he had logged 288.5 hours.

Erin woke up late, her lupus making her tired as usual and started the coffee. It was another day without Paul. It had been four days and she hadn't seen him at all, but that didn't mean she stopped her routine. After getting dressed for the cold weather and finishing her last sips of coffee she said,

"Come on you monkeys, you wanna go for a walk?" Her two best friends, her Basset Hounds Frederick Longfellow and Lilly Nelson, wagged their tails in excitement when they heard the word "walk." As she strolled with her "monkeys" along the beach and the wind whipped her hair into her face, she wondered what Paul was doing at this moment.

Beat down, cold, and exhausted Paul would go home for 6-10 hours once a week and sleep. The one day off a week minimum for every 10 days worked would also be set aside for rest. He wasn't much fun when he came home and he knew it. Erin didn't complain though. She knew he was doing this for her. The one thing that kept her going was the knowledge that in two months they would be together 24/7.

Paul never stops working toward the same goal. Even as he can't feel the tips off his fingers in the freezing cold temperatures, 5 to 15 degrees outside with negative wind chills, and working outside in what seems to be a continuous string of one snowstorm after another he perseveres. It's not just for him; it's for his wife Erin. He wants to give her something she thought she lost forever when she was hospitalized ten years ago. To live life again. To find the adventures and take them on together as a team. They were good at that. Paul needed it as much as she did. So he didn't give up. He worked.

****

Paul is all about the details. For months he has been a living Excel spreadsheet, categorizing different aspects of the trip.

He scoured craigslist, message boards, and dealers before running into the perfect black truck at a local dealer that had a buy here pay here policy. They shelled out $12,500 cash. With an original budget of $20,000 they had enough lee-way for repairs.

Paul was also in charge of the schedule. Erin and he shared a text file that read:

May: south va/tenn/mo

June: Iowa

July: Colorado/Utah

August: Washington/Oregon

Sept:calif

Oct: Las Vegas

Nov: Lake Havasu ??

Dec: Quartzsite

Jan: Quartzsite

Feb: Quartzsite

March: Florida

April - August: NJ/Pottsville

Sept-oct: Roscoe

On the phone Erin sounded most excited about Quartzsite.

"It's the largest deposit of quartz crystals in country. It's the largest RV meet up in the country! Thousands of people come there and set up shop. If you make jewelry you sell jewelry. It's like a flea market."

Over the phone, when I asked Erin if she was afraid of a lupus flare while on the road she said she wasn't.

"I'm over being afraid. If I was afraid I wouldn't be doing this trip. Plus, I trust Paul to have my back. He doesn't let me overdo it. When I'm in a flare he makes sure I take my medicine; he's always there to catch me. I'm over being scared for myself."

Erin and Paul can't have children. They made the decision that Erin take a medication that could make her sterile because there was no other option. She was too sick. Even if was possible for her to bear children, Erin says she would not because it wouldn't be fair for the baby.

"I think because of my body's history I wouldn't think my body would produce a healthy baby. I don't think it would be right or fair to the baby," she said.

Maybe that is one reason for taking a year off from everything and living in a camper as they travel the United States. But there is more than just no kids that is driving this drastic change of scenery.

Am I going to die, was a question that rose in Erin's mind many times when she first got sick. Ever since she's had to live under the shadow of lupus, never able to pursue her true dreams, never able to live the life she planned for herself. Her view of life is different from most of ours. When her father was diagnosed with a chronic illness, she knew how to relate to him at her young age of 35. She also thought he was given 60 good years. That's 60 good healthy years that she would have given anything to have. It made her contemplate things a bit more. You never know when life alters your course as it did to her ten years ago, and as it did to her dad.

"I'm sick now. I can't wait for retirement. We have to do something now," Erin said.

I can't think of a better way to do something. Think of all the people you've heard say, "I want to take a cross country road trip." Now think of all the people who actually do it. The investment to take on such a trip is immense. They had to save somewhere in the range of $30,000 dollars to see this adventure through. Add to that Erin's situation with lupus. Besides packing all her meds and her wheelchair for when a flare gets really bad, she'll need to set up doctors across the country that she can see in a pinch and who can communicate with her rheumatologist back home.

I asked Paul if he was afraid of Erin getting sick during the trip. Her getting sick during the trip did not make him most afraid. It was her never having the opportunity to take this trip in the first place that scared him the most.

"What am I afraid of the most with Erin? Very simple. I'm afraid of her dying prior to living a fulfilling life and without getting out there and living. Actually living," Paul wrote in an email to me. "Not living to make others happy or trying to live up to people's expectations of her, but living how she/we want to live, without regret. Seeing the mountains, seeing weird stuff like the world's biggest ball of yarn. So yes in a way this trip represents a lot. This trip is our insurance against the questions that most people either try to avoid or never think to ask themselves. What if I don't live to be 65? What if my spouse dies before then?"

****

I pulled up and there was a 35 foot camper parked on the other side of the street – the camper that Erin would call home for the next year of her life. Erin came to the front door of her parents' house to greet me and I hugged her as old friends. It was a going away party with all of Erin's family and friends. I met her mom Stacy and her dad Allan.

"You must be so proud of Erin," I said to Allan.

"Yes. She really deserves this," he said.

Deserves this. I couldn't agree more. Here I sat in the house where Erin stayed for one year, unable to walk. Yes, she deserves this.

A week ago Erin was putting what she didn't need for the trip into storage. That same day on Tuesday at 11 o'clock Stefania met with Jun preparing to submit their findings on TREX-1 to a journal for publication. On Saturday Paul Gallo decided to go in to the lab and collect urine from lupus prone mice. Meanwhile Erin "yarn bombed" a telephone pole near their rented home in Brigantine, NJ. She wrapped the pole with different color yarn from her knitting supplies to leave her mark on the town she called home. She sent a picture to me that said, "I even yarn bombed Brigantine!" Stefania and her lab work every day so that people like Erin can live how they want to live. Erin is proof of their efforts.

At the end of the night, filled to the brim with Stacy's food I sipped decaf at the kitchen table. In the corner of the table was my manuscript. Talking to Erin on the phone, in person, and over dinner had ended in what began as a school project. Six months later it morphed into so much more. It was Erin's inner most thoughts written in her diary late at night after combating her disease. It was my hesitation on how to use what she told me in a way not to exploit her illness but help others understand it. And here it was a celebration of not giving in, of persevering and coming out on top.

I know that during this trip Erin will battle like she always does. I know that there will be days when she needs her cane and her chest feels like it's on fire. But I also know that both Erin and Paul will be for the first time in a long time not living in fear of her disease but living in spite of it.

# Reflection

When I first began this project the only thing I knew for certain was that I wanted to write creative nonfiction. I hadn't taken a course on it yet, (that would come during the fall semester of my last year), and I wasn't sure how to write creative nonfiction, but I knew I liked reading it. So I figured I'd take a stab at it. The next concern was what to write about. I toyed with different ideas, bouncing back and forth between a personal memoir to writing about American politics. Finally, one day at dinner my dad asked what ever happened to Dr. Stefania Gallucci, the research scientist I worked for ten years ago. I resolved that it was a good question. Whatever did happen to her or her research, I wondered. Then I had my idea for a creative nonfiction piece. I thought I would write about the disease lupus and the different people who work on finding a cure.

My first day back at the lab I took pictures and notes on everything. In my phone are eight photographs of a poster that hung on the lab refrigerator. It was highly scientific saying, "In systemic lupus erythematosus virus-derived as well as endogenous (i.e. dsDNA, snRPs) nucleic acids can trigger Type I IFN secretion from pDCs." Now, I knew what that meant and I knew how to write it so that other biologists knew what it meant, but what was extremely difficult was to write it so that the general public knew what it meant. I employed different techniques to achieve this goal. For starters I used similes. For this sentence I might have said something like, "in lupus, DNA from outside invaders like viruses or necrotic cells, like cells that have been murdered, can cause dendritic cells to produce Type I Interferon. Type I Interferon is like the man in the watch tower yelling 'red alert' to start the immune response in the body."

I also employed another technique, and tried attempting to create a scene. Instead of simply saying Stefania worked on dendritic cells and found that endogenous signals can start the immune response in dendritic cells I wrote something like, "Stefania took a deceased mouse, as she had done thousands of times before and removed muscle tissue from the femur and the tibia. She cut both ends of the bone with scissors and then flushed out the bone marrow using a syringe. Stefania was used to this procedure. The push and the pull of the syringe almost had a rhythm to it."

Dr. Itzkowtiz, my second reader, suggested a book by surgeon Richard Selzer called *Mortal Lesson Notes on the Art of Surgery*. In it, Selzer writes about all the bodily systems, but he writes almost poetically. For example, he writes in the chapter titled "Bone," "Bones. Two hundred and eight of them. A whole glory turned and tooled. Lo the timbered femur all hung and strapped with beef, whose globate head nuzzles the concave underpart of the pelvis; the little carpals of the wrist faceted as jewels." I tried to similarly write in a literary fashion at some points. I tried to spice up a rather dry topic of the kidney with, "the kidney is the size of a large orange and in such high demand that 106,000 Americans wait for one each year. It looks like the bean that bears its name. Place your hands on your hips and your thumbs that extend around to the back are touching the pair of them. The kidney, that small but fierce organ, is an underappreciated hero. Everyone always pays homage to the heart, but the kidneys are the powerhouse, the workhorse of the body and without them you're as good as dead."

As I continued to write about the science, I soon realized I needed the view point of a patient. I needed a more human aspect to this story to make it affect the reader. I first met Erin Castaldi through an old high school acquaintance. I wasn't sure what to expect or if she would want me to write about her at all. It became pretty clear pretty quickly, however, that she was extremely open to the idea. What began as a first meeting at a coffee shop, developed into brunch, dinner, telephone conversations, emails and just hanging out. She let me delve into her mind and what it felt like to be plagued by a chronic illness like lupus. As I continued to write about Stefania and the lab I also began incorporating Erin into the story. I would say that looking at my project as a whole, Erin became one of the central 'characters' in the piece.

Erin and I had many interactions over the past six months. I think that is one aspect of this story I would like to explore further going forward. She trusted me enough to let me read seven of her diaries and pick quotes for the piece. I'd like to show a bit more that relationship that grew between us and my goal of not exploiting her but rather truthfully sharing her story.

Something about that really hit home when I went to her going away party this past weekend. Erin came up to me toward the end of the night as I was drinking my decaf coffee, and said that her mom, Stacy, had just started reading my manuscript today.

"She hasn't really said much to me since," Erin said to me.

My heard sank as I thought maybe I wrote something wrong or disparaged the family in some way, but Erin said no, it was just a difficult thing for her to read. I thought about the first few lines to the piece, "She felt like a spec. An inconsequential spec. What could she offer anyone? She couldn't even offer anything to herself. She was just another sick person, living off of government help because she couldn't afford the medication that only slightly lessened the pain she was in. She felt guilty. Guilty about not being a better wife. Guilty about needing government assistance. Guilty about not being a better citizen and not giving back anything to society. She viewed herself as a taker and she wanted so bad to be a giver." I realized those were Erin's words, I didn't embellish the truth, as so many literary journalists warn against. I also realized that it must be hard to read as a mother of a child that suffered so much. What hit me the hardest was these were real people with real lives that I wrote about and I wanted nothing more than to do them justice. I hope that this story does that. I hope that it opens the readers' eyes to just what it's like living with an illness. Even with an army of scientists working on a cure every day, it happens in small steps. They are heroes, both the patients like Erin and the researchers like Stefania.

.